Physiological Testing of the Elite Athlete

Edited by

J. Duncan MacDougall
Howard A. Wenger
Howard J. Green

D1501301

Published by
The Canadian Association of Sport Sciences
in collaboration with
The Sport Medicine Council of Canada

Canadian Cataloguing in Publication Data

Main entry under title:
Physiological testing of the elite athlete

Includes bibliographies and index.
ISBN 0-9691374-0-0

1. Athletic ability. 2. Physical fitness — Testing.
3. Sports — Physiological aspects. I. MacDougall, J. Duncan.
II. Wenger, Howard A. (Howard Allan).
III. Green, Howard J. IV. Canadian Association of
Sport sciences. V. Sport Medicine Council of Canada.

GV436.P49 1983 2   613.71   C83-099003-8

GV
436
.P49
1982

Printed in Canada by Mutual Press Limited.

Physiological Testing of the Elite Athlete

Edited by
J. Duncan MacDougall, Ph.D.
Departments of Physical Education and Medicine
McMaster University
Hamilton, Ontario

Howard A. Wenger, Ph.D.
School of Physical Education
University of Victoria
Victoria, British Columbia

Howard J. Green, Ph.D.
Department of Kinesiology
University of Waterloo
Waterloo, Ontario

The programs of this association are financially supported by **Sport Canada**

Les programmes de cette association reçoivent l'appui financier de **Sport Canada**

 Government of Canada
Fitness and Amateur Sport

Gouvernement du Canada
Condition physique et Sport amateur

MAJOR CONTRIBUTORS

Richard Backus, M.D.
  University of Victoria, Victoria, British Columbia.

Eric W. Banister, Ph.D.
  Department of Kinesiology, Simon Fraser University, Burnaby, British Columbia.

Claude Bouchard, Ph.D.
  Département d'éducation physique, Université Laval, Ste-Foy, Québec.

Serge Dulac, Ph.D.
  Département des sciences de l'activité physique, Université du Québec
  à Trois-Rivières, Trois-Rivières, Québec.

Howard J. Green, Ph.D.
  Department of Kinesiology, University of Waterloo, Waterloo, Ontario.

Cheryl Hubley, M.Sc.
  School of Physiotherapy, Dalhousie University, Halifax, Nova Scotia.

J. Duncan MacDougall, Ph.D.
  Departments of Physical Education and Medicine, McMaster University,
  Hamilton, Ontario.

Michael J. Marfell-Jones, Ph.D.
  Department of Kinesiology, Simon Fraser University, Burnaby, British Columbia.

Robert W. Norman, Ph.D.
  Department of Kinesiology, University of Waterloo, Waterloo, Ontario.

Alfred Reed, Ph.D.
  Department of Kinanthropology, University of Ottawa, Ottawa, Ontario.

William D. Ross, Ph.D.
  Department of Kinesiology, Simon Fraser University, Burnaby, British Columbia.

Digby G. Sale, Ph.D.
  Department of Physical Education, McMaster University, Hamilton, Ontario.

Albert W. Taylor, Ph.D.
  Département d'éducation physique, Université de Montréal, Montréal, Québec.

James S. Thoden, Ph.D.
  School of Human Kinetics, University of Ottawa, Ottawa, Ontario.

Howard A. Wenger, Ph.D.
  School of Physical Education, University of Victoria, Victoria, British Columbia.

Brian A. Wilson, Ph.D.
  School of Human Biology, University of Guelph, Guelph, Ontario.

FOREWORD

Through the efforts of agencies such as the Coaching Association of Canada, coaching and technical personnel are becoming increasingly aware of the importance of involving the sport scientist in the total preparation of the athlete. As a result, since the early 1970's, Canadian scientists have received more and more requests from both national and provincial sport governing bodies to conduct laboratory evaluations of their elite athletes.

During the 1979 general meeting of the Canadian Association of Sport Sciences in Vancouver and after a survey conducted by the Sport Medicine Council of Canada in 1980, it became obvious that many athlete-testing programs were failing to accomplish their objectives. The major criticisms were that —

1. the test batteries tended to be comprised of general tests of fitness which were not tailored to suit the specific needs of the elite athlete;

2. the coaches and athletes were unable to interpret properly the test results;

3. in certain instances, data had been collected for research purposes only and was of no direct assistance to the athletes; and

4. specific testing protocols varied from test to test and between laboratories to the extent that it was impossible to compare the results of one athlete with those of another.

Because of these concerns, the Canadian Association of Sport Sciences accepted the responsibility for developing a series of guidelines for the evaluation of the elite athlete. The present manual, which deals only with physiological testing, attempts to outline the potential importance of a proper testing program, and suggests appropriate tests and standardized protocols for their administration. It is intended for use by all coaches and technical directors as well as by those technicians and scientists who are involved with the testing and counselling of elite athletes.

The manual devotes a chapter to the evaluation of each of strength, flexibility, aerobic power, anaerobic power, and body composition and anthropometry. Each chapter includes the rationale for testing that particular component, its relevance to various sports, the validity and reliability of the testing procedures, guidelines for interpreting the results, and a suggested fee structure for administering the tests. The pages containing the test protocols for each chapter have been identified with tabs for rapid reference. In addition, there are chapters on evaluating the health status of the elite athlete, the use of field tests, and a summary of how test results can be used in order to monitor training progress. An underlying theme throughout the manual is that test items must be sport-specific. It is therefore intended that, in many instances, the protocols which have been suggested must be modified to meet the needs of an individual sport.

The authors who have contributed to this manual not only are knowledgeable scientists in their fields but also have considerable experience in the laboratory testing of athletes. In addition to their efforts, we wish to acknowledge the valuable advice and assistance of the Sport Medicine Council of Canada and of Pat Reid and Jim Shaw of Sport Canada. We also thank Pauline McCullagh, Project Manager, Laura Diskin, Secretarial Assistant, and Diane M. Kerss, Advisor.

D. MacDougall
H. Wenger
H. Green

CONTENTS

The Purpose of Physiological Testing

J.D. MacDougall • H.A. Wenger

INTRODUCTION

The superior performances of today's athletes are the result of a complex blend of many physiological, biomechanical, and psychological factors. The modern coach recognizes that the most consistently effective method of preparing his athletes for competition is one which is based on proven scientific principles rather than on trial and error or on empirical judgment. It is therefore becoming more and more common for the coach and the athlete to seek input from the sport scientist in order that the athlete be enabled to achieve his full potential.

What the Athlete Gains

An ongoing program of properly selected and administered laboratory tests can become an expensive and time consuming process and the question arises as to whether or not the returns can justify the investment. An effective testing program is of benefit to the athlete and coach in several ways:

1. *It indicates the athlete's strengths and weaknesses, relevant to his sport, and provides baseline data for individual training program prescription.* Most sports and activities involve several physiological components. Although in the field setting it may be relatively easy to evaluate the sum result, it usually is difficult to assess the athlete on each of the individual components. In the laboratory, the scientist is often able to isolate a given component and to assess objectively the athlete's performance on that variable. These results then become the basis for prescribing an optimal training program and one which can concentrate on identified areas of weakness.

2. *It provides feedback for evaluating the effectiveness of a given training program.* Comparison of an individual's results on a given test item with those of his previous tests provides a basis for assessing the effectiveness of the intervening program. Moreover, the coach may find that a program which proves effective for one athlete may be less effective for another. The results of a valid test for that variable will confirm this.

3. *It provides information as to the health status of the athlete.* Training for high level competition is a physically demanding and stressful procedure which may in itself create health problems in the athlete. Moreover, the fact that an individual is an athlete does not necessarily ensure that he is free from disease. Special measures as outlined in Chapter 9, in addition to certain performance tests, may sometimes reveal abnormalities which might not be detected by a standard physical examination.

4. *It is an educational process by which the athlete learns to understand better his body and the demands of his sport.* The process of interpreting test results to the athlete becomes a medium by which the athlete can increase his understanding of the physiological components of his sport as well as his own body awareness.

What Testing Will Not Do

Laboratory testing is not a magical tool for predicting future gold medalists. It has severe limitations for identifying potential talent in that scientists still do not know how to determine "genetic limits" and therefore cannot predict potential to improve. For example, the use of muscle biopsies to estimate muscle fiber types and thus predict endurance or power performance is highly questionable, first, because a single biopsy is a poor predictor of the whole muscle make-up (Elder et al., 1982), and second, because there is substantial overlap in the fiber type profiles of elite endurance and power athletes.

The complete performance of any athlete is a composite of many different factors of which physiological function is only one. It is therefore unwise to attempt to predict performance from any single physiological test or battery of physiological tests — especially in sports where technical, tactical, and psychological components may relegate physiology to a lesser role. Similarly, in the selection of athletes for competition or for teams, physiological tests should only augment information which is available on actual performances or field observations.

What Constitutes an Effective Testing Program

An effective testing program is one where —

1. *the variables which are tested are relevant to that sport.* Although this might appear to be an obvious statement, it has not been unusual in the past for the coach, athlete, and scientist to have wasted considerable time by testing physiological components which have little application to their particular sport or its problems.

2. *the tests which are selected are valid and reliable.* A test is valid when it actually measures what it claims to measure. It is reliable when the results are consistent and reproducible. The scientist may administer what he considers to be a valid test, but if the reliability of the test is not sufficiently high to reflect the slight changes which might occur in the elite athlete over a given training period, it is of little value.

3. *the test protocols are as sport-specific as possible.* For the test results to have optimum practical significance, the exercise mode must be specific to the sport. For example, a maximal aerobic or anaerobic capacity test which uses a treadmill-running protocol, when administered to a swimmer, will give very little information regarding his state of training for swimming. Ideally, he should be tested in a swimming flume, or "swimming treadmill". Since such a facility does not yet exist in Canada, the next best choice is to test him on a simulated swimming task, such as arm-ergometry, tethered swimming, or exercise on a swim bench. In such cases, despite the fact that results may be highly reliable, their validity declines as the motor pattern becomes more and more removed from that of swimming.

4. *test administration is rigidly controlled.* Once test items are selected, they must be administered consistently at all times. This necessitates standard instructions to the athletes, standard practice or warm-up procedures, standard order of test items and recovery time between items, standard environmental temperature and humidity, and standard equipment and equipment calibration procedures. In addition, all intra-athlete variables which might affect test results should be carefully recorded. These include details such as the stage of training, the time of the most recent competition, the time of day in relation to previous tests, the nutritional status of the athlete, and other interventions such as sleep, injury or illness, hydration, drugs, or anxiety.

5. *the athlete's human rights are respected.* Ethical criteria which must be met before administering a test include: a thorough explanation of the purpose of the test; a realistic statement of the possible physical or psychological risks involved in the test; and provision for ensuring that confidentiality of test results will be maintained. (For a sample Informed Consent Form see Appendix 4.1, Chapter 4.)

6. *testing is repeated at regular intervals.* Since one of the main purposes of testing is to monitor training effectiveness, it is apparent that the tests must be repeated following different phases of training. "One-shot" testing, or even once-per-year testing, although of potential interest to the scientist, is of little practical value to the athlete.

7. *results are interpreted to the coach and athlete directly.* This final, crucial step often is the one which is most poorly handled by the scientist. Not only must test results be reported promptly to the athlete, but also they must be interpreted in language which he and his coach understand.

REFERENCE

Elder, G.C.B., K. Bradbury, and R. Roberts. Variability of fiber type distribution within human muscles. *J. Appl. Physiol.: Respirat. Environ, Exercise Physiol.* 53(6): 1473-80, 1982.

TWO

Overview of the Energy Delivery Systems

H.J. Green

INTRODUCTION

In elite sport, the ultimate concern is with the final performance, whether such performance occurs in shotputting, wrestling, distance running, or archery. The final output that we observe, however, is dependent upon a complexity of factors, each of which may contribute a variable amount to the performance. Tests allow the measurement of specific fundamental factors, assumed to be important in that performance. These factors can then be evaluated and appropriate training strategies developed to provide for the improvement of any weak links.

The output of the human machine can be defined in physical quantities such as work, power, and force. The output that is measured is ultimately dependent on the muscle or muscles involved in the activity. Since muscles act over joints, however, and since different lever systems and joint angles are involved, mechanical factors must also be considered. If extrapolations are to be made to the physical potential of a particular muscle or muscle group, the mechanical factors must be identified and controlled.

Measurement of Muscular Force and Power

Tests of muscular force and power attempt to evaluate the contractile activity occurring in specific muscles. The total potential contractile activity is limited by the number and size of the muscle fibers. Similarly, the percentage utilization of the muscle fiber pool at any one time during voluntary activity is dependent on both neural and energetic considerations. For the voluntary output to approach the maximal capability, not only must all fibers be recruited, but the firing frequency of each motor unit, and the synchronization of the firing pattern between motor units must be optimal (Figure 2.1). In addition, not only must the chemical energy, ATP, be present in non-limiting amounts, but the rate of breakdown of the ATP to provide the energy for contraction must not be limiting. If either of these processes is restrictive, the force or power value obtained will not represent the contractile potential of the muscle.

The standardization of test protocols in this area involves defining the body and limb position so that the performance of a particular muscle can be isolated. In addition, both angle of measurement and velocity of movement must be specified carefully, since both of these factors influence force and power determinations. Also, since specific neural co-ordination patterns are involved, tests must attempt to minimize the learning factor by allowing sufficient practice trials.

The rigorous standardization procedures necessary for objective measurement in this area mean that only a very specific behaviour of muscle function is evaluated. For such tests to have applicability to sport performances, they must reflect as closely as possible the manner in which the muscle or muscle groups are employed.

Measurement of Energy Potential

Sources of Chemical Energy

For muscle contraction to occur, chemical energy in the form of Adenosine Triphosphate (ATP) must be available. Since ATP is in very low concentration in the muscle, and since it decreases only to a minor extent, even in the most intense voluntary contraction, tightly controlled mechanisms must exist for the continual regeneration of ATP as contraction continues.

The mechanisms (chemical pathways) for regeneration of ATP involve three distinct processes.

1. *Creatine Phosphate Splitting.* Creatine Phosphate (CP) is a high energy phosphagen

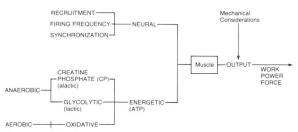

Fig. 2.1   Neural and energetic processes involved in muscle performance.

similar to ATP. In skeletal muscle, this compound has a concentration approximately three-fold greater than ATP. One of its functions is to regenerate the ATP that has been broken down during contraction. Creatine Phosphate is particularly important as a source of ATP regeneration early in intense exercise where greater than 80% depletion has been observed. The high energy phosphagens, ATP and CP, have been referred to as *alactic anaerobic* energy sources. This term emphasizes the facts that oxygen is not used directly (anaerobic) and lactic acid is not formed (alactic).

CP is extremely limited in its ability to regenerate large amounts of ATP. Beyond the first several seconds of intense exercise, other metabolic pathways must predominate if ATP levels are to remain high. These pathways include aerobic (oxidative) and anaerobic (glycolytic) processes (see Figure 2.2).

2. *Aerobic (Oxidative) Metabolism.* The production of ATP by aerobic processes involves the combustion of a fuel in the muscle cell in the presence of oxygen. The fuel can come from sources within the muscle (free fatty acids, glycogen) and from sources outside the muscle (free fatty acids from adipose tissue, glucose from the liver). For this type of metabolism to contribute significantly, oxygen must be supplied to the mitochondria in the muscle cells in appropriate amounts. Since the oxygen comes from the atmosphere, respiratory and cardiovascular processes must be capable of taking up and delivering large volumes of oxygen. The by-products of aerobic metabolism are water and carbon dioxide. The water is partially retained in the body to assist in maintaining homeostasis; carbon dioxide is eliminated to the atmosphere.

3. *Anaerobic Glycolysis.* The regeneration of ATP through anaerobic glycolysis involves the breakdown of carbohydrate (mainly muscle gly-

cogen) to lactic acid. Since oxygen is not used and since lactic acid is formed, this source of ATP is described also as *anaerobic lactic*. Although large amounts of ATP can be regenerated from this energy pathway per unit time, it is not possible to continue contraction for prolonged periods using glycolytic processes. The large acidosis resulting from lactic acid accumulation and/or the rapid rate of glycogen depletion ultimately forces a reduction in work intensity.

In summary, the measurement of energy potential of the muscle involves the measurement of three distinct metabolic processes that form the basis of ATP regeneration in exercise. These processes include anaerobic mechanisms (glycolytic and high energy phosphagens) and aerobic mechanisms (oxygen).

In connection with these energy systems, a distinction must also be made between the *capacity* and *power* of each system. The total amount of ATP production from a given system relates to the capacity of that system. The maximal amount of ATP production occurring per unit time is referred to as the power of the system. In theory at least, six different components must be measured for a

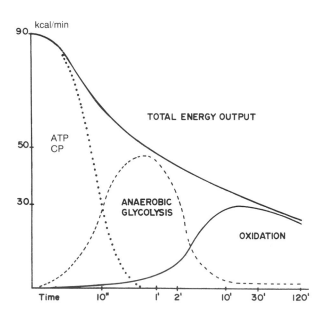

Fig. 2.2.   Sequence and quantitative relationships of energy-supplying biochemical processes in human skeletal muscle. The duration of exercise is given on a logarithmic scale and the energy outputs are calculated on the basis of results performed by top athletes in the different activities concerned. (From Howald, von Glutz, and Billeter, 1978)

comprehensive evaluation of the energy potential of a muscle. These include the capacity and power of each of the three different energy metabolic processes.

UTILIZATION OF ENERGY SYSTEMS DURING EXERCISE

The three energy systems cannot be thought of as isolated processes which operate independently during exercise. Rather, they are integrated and operate in concert so that the supply of ATP can be altered in an attempt to satisfy the energy requirements of the muscle. All three processes occur concurrently; the proportion, however, of ATP supplied from each process will vary according to the intensity and duration of the exercise.

Under normal resting conditions, most of the ATP in skeletal muscle is regenerated via aerobic processes at a rate which matches its rate of utilization. A rapid increase in exercise intensity is accommodated by an accelerated rate of alactic generation of ATP (mainly CP) and anaerobic glycolysis (lactic generation of ATP) followed by a more gradual acceleration of aerobic metabolism. If the rate of ATP utilization can eventually be matched by aerobic regeneration, the contributions of the other two systems will be proportionately reduced, resulting in relatively stable levels of muscle and plasma lactic acid. If, however, the intensity of the activity is extremely high, the anaerobic systems will continue to represent a major source of ATP. This occurs because peak ability of the aerobic processes to supply ATP is considerably below the energy demands of the muscle.

The contribution of the various energy sources over time during maximal activity is represented in Figure 2.2 and Table 2.1. As can be seen, there is a rapid drop-off in muscle performance and consequently in the energy utilization by the muscle over time. During short work periods (less than two minutes) when the ATP utilization is high, the energy source is primarily anaerobic. As the exercise is extended, the aerobic sources contribute an increasing proportion. This occurs because the oxidative pathway has been accelerated to peak potential and because the energy utilization of the muscle has been greatly reduced.

Most tests designed to measure the characteristics of the energy system, then, are time dependent. The assumption is that, by using tests of different durations, the contribution of a particular

energy source will be maximized and the effect of the others will be minimized. Consequently, the performance that is measured should reflect the potential of the particular energy system in question.

Table 2.1 The energy delivery systems in terms of performance time, with examples of physical activities*

MAJOR ENERGY SYSTEMS	PERFORMANCE TIME	EXAMPLES OF TYPE OF PHYSICAL ACTIVITIES
ATP and CP	Less than 20 seconds	Shot-put, 100-meter sprint, base stealing, golf and tennis swings, running plays of football backs
ATP and CP and Anaerobic Glycolysis (Lactic acid)	From about 30 seconds to 90 seconds	200- to 400-meter sprints, speed skating, 100-meter swim
Anaerobic Glycolysis (Lactic acid) and Aerobic	From about 90 seconds to several minutes	800-meter dash, gymnastics events, boxing (3-min. rounds), wrestling (2-min. periods)
Aerobic	More than several minutes	Soccer and lacrosse (except goalies), cross-country skiing, marathon run, jogging

*Modified from Fox, 1979

CONSIDERATIONS IN MEASUREMENT OF STRENGTH, POWER, AND ENERGY POTENTIAL

The measurement of the output of a system can be defined in physical terms such as force, power, and work. Theoretically, each muscle cell can be categorized as having specific values for each of these physical parameters. In addition, each muscle cell can be characterized as having a specific aerobic and anaerobic energy potential. In practice, however, measurements are made on a particular muscle, or group of muscles, acting over one or two joints. Consequently, the calculation of the physical output of the muscle (and the energy potential) must consider also the mechanical factors involved. In tests involving force and power outputs, body position and joint angle must be rigidly standardized so that the test value measures the specific muscle, or muscle groups, in question.

In such tests, the contractile activity of the muscle must be relatively brief, thereby permitting the energy to be supplied exclusively from the high energy phosphagens. In voluntary performance of this nature, the force and/or power characteristics reflect the summated contractile activity occurring in the muscle during the test. The amount of contractile activity may reflect not only the number of contractile elements in the muscle (muscle fibers) but also the neural recruitment pattern and the rate at which energy can be supplied by the splitting of ATP.

Although the measurement of the energy potential theoretically should be standardized to specific muscles, such generally has not been the case. Rather, groups of muscles (especially those of locomotion) are commonly employed to test for aerobic and anaerobic capabilities. In the case of the aerobic system, measurement of *aerobic power* has been used almost exclusively. Such tests have employed large muscle groups (involved in running, cycling, and swimming) and have measured directly the peak oxygen utilized per unit time (see Chapter 4). There is no agreement at this time as to whether the aerobic power that is obtained is limited by the uptake and delivery of oxygen to the working muscles, or by the collective oxidative metabolic processes of the contracting muscles.

Similarly, the measurement of anaerobic energy characteristics generally has not been restricted to isolated muscle groups. Rather, it has been calculated on performance-based tests involving the co-ordination of a number of muscles and joints. The measurements obtained must be interpreted accordingly.

In conclusion, measurement of force, power, or energy potential depends on careful standardization of test protocols. The test procedures must be founded on objective and scientifically verified criteria. Since most of these parameters are muscle specific, they must be interpreted with caution when evaluated in the context of a specific sport behaviour. Unquestionably, the degree to which a test will be valid will depend on a close simulation of the test with the movements occurring in the sport. Test development must be viewed as an ongoing process. Refinement can occur only through a constant dialogue between the coach, the athlete, and the scientist.

REFERENCES

Fox, E.L. *Sports Physiology,* Saunders, Philadelphia, 1979.

Howald, H., G. von Glutz and R. Billeter. Energy stores and substrates utilization in muscle during exercise, in *The Third International Symposium on Biochemistry of Exercise.* F. Landry and W.A.R. Orban (eds.), Miami Symposia Specialists, 1978, pp. 75-86.

CHAPTER THREE

Testing Strength and Power

D.G. Sale • R.W. Norman
with contributions from D.A. Dainty

INTRODUCTION

Definitions

Strength is usually defined as the peak force or torque developed during a maximal voluntary contraction (MVC). The SI (the abbreviation for *Système international d'unités*, the International System of Units) units for force and torque are the newton (N) and newton meter (N·m), respectively. The weight of a one kilogram (kg) mass (2.2 lb) is 9.80665 N (9.8 N for short!).

Power (P) is defined as the time (t) rate at which mechanical work (W) is performed; thus, $P = W/t$ or $W \times t^{-1}$. Power may also be expressed as the product of force (F) and velocity (V); thus, $P = F \times V$. The SI unit for power is the watt (W). A power of 1.0 W would occur when work was performed at a rate of one joule per second (J/s), which is the same as a force of 1.0 N acting at a velocity of 1.0 m/s (or a torque of 1.0 N·m acting at a velocity of 1 rad/s). Additional information on units of measurement will be presented below in the section *Units of Measurement*.

Effect of Contraction Type and Contraction Velocity Upon Peak Force and Torque

There are three types of muscle contraction: (1) *isometric* — in which the muscle length remains unchanged while producing tension; (2) *concentric* — in which the muscle shortens while producing tension; (3) *eccentric* — in which the muscle lengthens while producing tension. Of these three contraction types, eccentric contractions are the strongest and concentric contractions are the weakest. In the case of concentric and eccentric contractions, the peak force of maximal contractions is affected also by the velocity of shortening and lengthening respectively. An increase in the velocity of shortening causes a decrease in the force of concentric contractions,

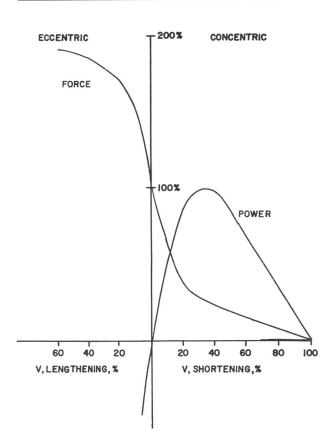

Fig. 3.1 Effect of velocity and contraction type upon muscle force and power. In concentric contractions, force decreases with increased velocity of shortening. In eccentric contractions, force increases with increased velocity of lengthening. On the ordinate, 100% represents maximum isometric force and maximum power of concentric contractions. In concentric contractions, the velocity at which peak power occurs will vary but is usually less than 50% of the maximal velocity.

while an increase in the velocity of lengthening causes, up to a point, an increase in the force of eccentric contractions. Figure 3.1 illustrates the effects of contraction type and velocity upon the force of muscle contractions. The effects of contraction type and velocity upon contraction force are not related to variations in motor unit activation (Komi, 1973; Rodgers and Berger, 1974) or metabolism (Komi and Viitasalo, 1977), but rather to variations in the interaction of the myosin and actin filaments within the myofibrils of muscle fibers (for a contrary view on the effect of velocity on motor unit activation during concentric contractions, see Nelson et al., 1973 and Barnes, 1980).

The effects of contraction type and velocity upon power are illustrated also in Figure 3.1. In isometric contractions, the power is zero because the velocity is zero ($P = F \times V$). In concentric contractions, the velocity at which greatest power occurs varies but is usually less than 50% of the maximal shortening velocity. Above the velocity at which peak power occurs, the power declines and becomes zero when the force is zero at the maximal shortening velocity. In eccentric contractions, the muscle absorbs energy; that is, work is done against the muscle. The rate at which this work (energy) is absorbed (sometimes called negative work) is called the negative power. The negative power increases with increased velocity of eccentric contractions because both velocity and force are increasing.

The effects of contraction type and velocity upon muscle strength and power are striking. An understanding of these effects is helpful in the design and interpretation of strength tests. In particular, the test design should take into account the contraction type and velocity characteristics of the sport movements.

Effect of Muscle Length and Muscle Angle of Pull

The peak force which can be developed by a muscle or muscle group varies through a range of movement. This variation in peak force is called a "strength curve". Some examples of strength curves are illustrated in Figure 3.2. The shape of a strength curve is determined by two primary factors: (1) the length-tension effect; (2) the perpendicular distance between the line of pull of the muscle and the axis of the joint at which the muscle acts.

The length-tension effect refers to the variation

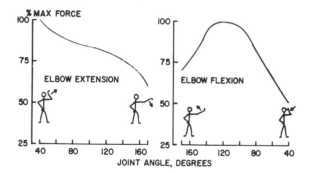

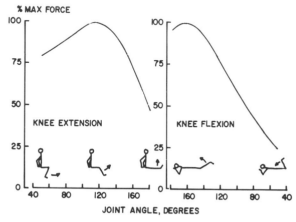

Fig. 3.2 Strength curves. The variation in voluntary muscle force through a range of movement for four movements is illustrated. Notice that the shape of the strength "curves" varies in the different movements. Based on Clarke (1966).

in contraction force that occurs when a muscle contracts at different muscle lengths. Generally, the contraction force is smallest at very short muscle lengths. The peak of the length-tension curve usually occurs at a length close to, or at, the longest possible muscle length when the muscle is intact in the body.

Muscles cause rotational movements at joints by producing torque. The magnitude of the torque produced depends upon the force of muscle contraction and the magnitude of the perpendicular distance between the "line of pull" of the muscle and the axis of the joint. The greater the perpendicular distance, the greater the torque produced for a given muscle force. The perpendicular distance between the line of pull of the muscle and the axis of the joint varies at different joint angles.

The shape of the strength curve for a range of movement at a joint is the resultant of the interaction and relative importance of the length-tension

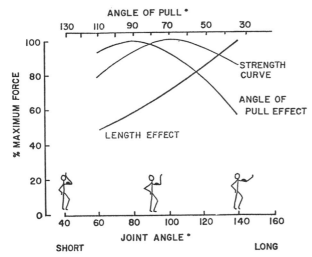

Fig. 3.3   Effect of muscle length and angle of pull upon elbow flexion strength. The length-tension effect and the angle of pull effect interact to produce the strength curve for elbow flexion. Through the range of movement depicted, the length effect acts to increase muscle tension from the shortest to longest muscle lengths. The longest length corresponds to an elbow joint angle (bottom horizontal axis) of 140°. In contrast the optimum angle of pull (90°, see top horizontal axis) occurs at a joint angle of about 80°. Thus, the peak of the resultant strength curve would be expected to occur somewhere between joint angles of 80° and 140°; in fact, it occurs at a joint angle of about 100°.

effect and the perpendicular distance effect. A hypothetical example of the interaction of these two factors in producing the strength curve for elbow flexion is presented in Figure 3.3.

A knowledge of strength curves and the variation in the force or torque which can be developed through a range of movement serves to emphasize the importance of standardizing and making consistent the joint position or range of movement used in strength tests.

Factors Affecting Strength Performance

Several characteristics of athletes will affect their strength performance. The interpretation of strength test results should take into consideration the influence of these characteristics, which will now be discussed briefly.

Muscle Size

There is a positive correlation between muscle cross-sectional area and absolute strength (Ikai

and Fukunaga, 1968). Thus, on the average, athletes with large muscles will be stronger than athletes with small muscles. There may be some exceptions to this general rule because of the other factors which affect strength performance. For example, an athlete with modest muscle size may still present a high strength performance if he/she possesses superior neural control of his/her muscles and if his/her muscles are inserted so as to provide a greater than normal mechanical advantage.

Body Size

The two most common ways of expressing the results of voluntary strength measurements are absolutely and in relation to body mass. Thus, an athlete with a body mass of 75 kg might have an absolute strength of 750 N·m in a test movement; the athlete's strength/mass ratio would be 10.0 N·m/kg.

There is a positive correlation between body size or body mass and absolute strength (Berger, 1982, p. 23). This correlation would be expected because a large body size is associated with a large muscle size. In contrast, there is a negative correlation between body size or mass and the strength/mass ratio (Berger, 1982, p. 23). Therefore, large athletes tend to have high absolute strength while small athletes tend to have a high strength/mass ratio. The results of world class weight lifting competitions illustrate well the effect of body mass on absolute strength and the strength/mass ratio, because the athletes are relatively homogeneous with respect to other factors which affect strength performance (Figure 3.4).

The foregoing explains why large athletes dominate sport events which require a high level of absolute strength (e.g., throwing events in track and field) and why small athletes dominate sport events which require a high strength/body mass ratio (e.g., gymnastics). There are some sport events which call for a compromise. For example, a high jumper needs a high strength/mass ratio but also needs to be tall. A high jumper whose height is 1.0 m would have to have a very high strength/mass ratio indeed to compensate for his/her short height! There are some sport events which require absolute strength in some movements and "relative" (strength/mass ratio) strength in others. In hockey, for example, the velocity of puck shooting and the execution of certain defensive maneuvers require absolute strength, while acceleration in

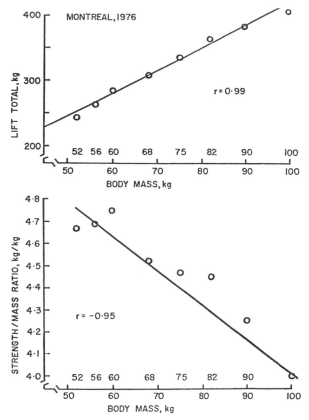

Fig. 3.4 Effect of body mass (size) on strength performance. Top: The winning Olympic (Montreal, 1976) weight lifting performances are presented for each body mass (weight) class. The vertical axis gives the total lifted for the two lifts (snatch and clean and jerk). The horizontal axis gives the body mass classes. Notice that greater lift totals were associated with a greater body mass. Thus, there was a positive correlation between absolute strength and body mass. Bottom: In contrast, there was a negative correlation between body mass and the strength/body mass ratio (vertical axis, total lifted divided by body mass); that is, the highest strength/body mass ratios were obtained by the "lightest" weight lifters.

skating requires relative strength. In hockey, therefore, athletes with a wide range in body size can be successful. Generally, when an external object is to be resisted or moved, absolute strength is most important; when the body mass itself is to be supported or moved, the strength/mass ratio is most important.

Muscle Fiber Composition

Human skeletal muscle is composed of two types of muscle fibers: (1) fast twitch (subtyped

into fast twitch glycolytic or IIB fibers and fast twitch glycolytic oxidative or IIA fibers) and (2) slow twitch fibers (slow twitch oxidative or I fibers). Human fast twitch fibers may be able to develop more force per unit cross-section area, as has been observed in animal muscle (Burke and Edgerton, 1975). This may explain the positive correlation that has been observed in humans between isometric strength and the percentage of fast twitch fibers (Tesch and Karlsson, 1978). Fast twitch fibers, however, are also able to develop force more rapidly; consequently, the correlation between the percentage of fast twitch fibers and strength becomes progressively stronger as strength is measured at progressively higher velocities (Coyle et al., 1979). Thus, athletes who possess a high proportion of fast twitch fibers in the relevant muscle groups should be at an advantage when the sport movement requires strong muscle contractions at high velocities. Perhaps unfortunately, fast twitch fibers have lesser resistance to fatigue than slow twitch fibers; therefore, a muscle with a high percentage of fast twitch fibers fatigues rapidly during high intensity exercise (Thorstensson and Karlsson, 1976).

Neural Factors

Voluntary strength performance depends not only upon the quantity and quality of muscle tissue, but also upon the ability of the nervous system to activate the muscle mass. There is evidence that under normal conditions many untrained individuals cannot fully activate their muscles (Ikai and Steinhaus, 1961). Special circumstances or training may enhance the ability to activate muscles. With respect to training, the degree to which motoneuron excitability can be raised during voluntary effort has been shown to be enhanced in elite sprinters (Upton and Radford, 1975) and weight lifters (Milner-Brown et al., 1975). Motor unit synchronization was enhanced in weight lifters and in those whose occupation involved making brief maximal contractions (Milner-Brown et al., 1975). The important role of the nervous system in strength performance is not surprising when it is considered that the expression of strength is in part a skilled act. Even when strength training involves a simple movement, there is evidence that the initial increases in voluntary strength are the result of neural rather than muscle adaptation (Moritani and deVries, 1979).

Age and Sex

In untrained males and females, peak absolute strength occurs in the mid-twenties; thereafter, it declines gradually; at age 65, about 80% of the peak strength is still retained (Fisher and Birren, 1947). When the results in many muscle groups are averaged, females possess approximately 60% of the absolute strength of males (Fisher and Birren, 1947). The gender difference in strength varies according to muscle group. In adults, females may possess 75% of the leg strength but only 50% of the arm-shoulder strength of males (Wilmore, 1974).

In males, the strength/body mass ratio peaks in the early twenties. In contrast, the strength/mass ratio in females may peak before puberty, particularly in the case of upper body strength (Montoye and Lamphiear, 1977).

The gender difference in strength is reduced when strength is expressed per kilogram body mass rather than absolutely, because males on the average have a greater body mass. When strength is expressed per kilogram lean body mass, the difference is further reduced, and there may be no difference in the case of leg strength (Anderson et al., 1979). This latter finding, combined with the observation that the strength per unit cross-sectional area is similar in males and females (Ikai and Fukunaga, 1968), suggests that the gender difference in strength is related to quantity rather than to quality of muscle tissue.

There is, however, some evidence that the male/female strength ratio is greater for high than for low velocity strength performance (Anderson et al., 1979), and that males can develop a given percentage of peak isometric force more rapidly than females (Komi and Karlsson, 1979). This difference in performance is not due to a greater proportion of fast twitch fibers in male muscle, but may be related to undefined neural mechanisms (Komi and Karlsson, 1978) or to a gender difference in muscle elasticity.

Trainability

There is abundant evidence that voluntary strength can be increased by appropriate training, and that in response to training there is adaptation within the muscles and the nervous system. It is also clear that the effects of strength training are very specific; the strength training exercises should simulate the sport movement patterns as closely as possible (Sale and MacDougall, 1981). The return on the training investment, in terms of the percentage increase in sport performance for a given percentage increase in strength as measured with the training device, will depend upon the degree to which the specificity principle has been applied in the training, and upon the relative importance of strength and power to the sport performance. For example, a group of sprint swimmers trained for one month on a very specific strength training machine. Strength measured on the machine increased by 19% while swim performance improved by 4% (Sharp et al., 1982). In cases where the training has been less specific, and/or strength and power are less important to performance, the transfer of training improvement to performance improvement will be even more modest.

Strength training sometimes results in a significant increase in muscle mass. An increase in muscle or body mass would not be desirable in an athlete whose sport requires a high strength/body mass ratio; strength training programs can be designed which minimize the increase in muscle or body mass (Sprague, 1979, p. 111). Fortunately, provided that the training is specific, the strength/body mass ratio usually increases after strength training even when there has been an increase in muscle mass. In a group of female athletes who performed strength training for six months, lean body mass increased but body fat decreased. There was no net increase in body mass, and the strength/mass ratio increased to the same degree as absolute strength (Brown and Wilmore, 1974). When the training causes an increase in body mass, the strength/mass ratio usually will still increase, because part of the training effect occurs in the nervous system and neural adaptation is "mass-free". In a shotputter whose training progress was monitored over a 5-year period, body mass increased by 34 kg (38%); the strength/mass ratio increased by 20%, however, because absolute strength had increased by 70%. The shotput performance increased by 5 m (31%) (O'Shea, 1969, p. 64). This case represents the upper limit of the range for body mass increase resulting from strength training; thus, almost all athletes can expect an increase in the strength/mass ratio despite any increase in body mass which is caused by an increase in muscle mass. What should be avoided is the development of irrelevant muscle groups, which would add to body mass but would not contribute to relevant strength.

RELEVANCE AND RELATIVE IMPORTANCE OF STRENGTH AND POWER TO SPORT PERFORMANCE

Variation in Relevance and Relative Importance

The relevance and relative importance of strength and power to sport performance will, of course, vary widely in different sports. There are several activities, such as weight lifting and the throwing, jumping, and sprinting events in track and field, in which strength and power are the dominating factors (after technique has been accounted for). There are also some activities in which strength and power would be relatively unimportant; examples are "pure" skill events (e.g., pistol shooting) and long duration endurance events (e.g., marathon running, long distance cross-country skiing, and long distance swimming). In most activities, however, (e.g., team sports, swimming, rowing, canoeing), strength and power share importance with endurance (see Chapters 4 and 5). In these activities, the actual relative importance of strength and endurance can be determined only by research; in fact, one of the purposes of strength and power testing may be to determine the relative importance of strength to a particular sport performance (see the section *PURPOSES OF TESTING STRENGTH AND POWER*, below). For example, maximal power was measured on a quasi-isokinetic "swim bench" and correlated with swimming velocity in a group of competitive swimmers. The correlations between power and swimming velocity were r = 0.90, r = 0.86, r = 0.85, and r = 0.76 for swim distances of 25 yd, 100 yd, 200 yd, and 500 yd, respectively (Sharp et al., 1982). As might be expected, as the swim distance increased, strength became less, and presumably endurance became more, important. Nevertheless, strength was an important factor in all distances, and over half the variation ($r^2 \times 100$) in swimming velocity was accounted for by the variation in specific strength.

Strength and Endurance

A high level of strength enhances short-term, high intensity "endurance", because a given absolute force or power output can be maintained longer when it represents a relatively smaller percentage of the maximum force or power capability. Thus, an athlete whose maximum strength was 1000 N would be able to sustain a force of 800 N, representing 80% of maximal strength, for 15 to 20 s, while an athlete whose maximum was 2000 N would be able to sustain 800 N, representing 40% of the maximum, for 2 to 3 min. This argument (Edington and Edgerton, 1976, p. 276) has most validity when the absolute load taxes a relatively high percentage of maximum strength and power; in this case, anaerobic metabolism limits performance. In long-term, low intensity exercise, performance is limited more by aerobic metabolism; in addition, large variations in strength do not cause large variations in the percentage of maximal strength which is taxed. In the example cited above, sustaining a force of 100 N would tax 10% of the strength of the weaker (max = 1000 N) athlete and 5% of the strength of the stronger (max = 2000 N) athlete. Compare this 5% difference in relative load (10% vs. 5%) with the 40% difference in relative load (80% vs. 40%) for the absolute load of 800 N.

It follows, therefore, that increasing strength by training would improve high, but probably not low, intensity endurance performance. Strength training may even impair endurance at low relative intensities for three reasons: (1) an increase in muscle mass and body mass would increase the energy requirement of activities involving support of the body mass; (2) strength training causes a decrease in mitochondrial volume density (MacDougall et al., 1979) which may decrease the oxidative capacity of the muscle; (3) strength training causes relatively greater hypertrophy of fast than slow twitch muscle fibers (Thorstensson et al., 1976; MacDougall et al., 1980). Thus, fast twitch fibers would contribute more to the increased strength, but their greater fatigability would reduce endurance with a given low relative load. These deleterious effects of strength training upon endurance performance can be attenuated by concurrent aerobic training, an approach followed by athletes whose sport performance requires both strength and endurance.

Strength and Speed

A high level of strength and power is usually associated with a greater ability to accelerate the body mass or external objects; the association is justified (Berger, 1982, p. 26). For example, an athlete for whom a load of 100 kg would tax 50% of maximum strength would be able to accelerate the load more than an athlete for whom the load represented 90% of maximum strength. When loads are normalized to represent the same percentage of maximum strength, the acceleration performance is similar in high and low strength individuals.

Therefore, an athlete with a high strength/body mass ratio would be more sucessful at accelerating the body mass in activities such as sprinting and jumping, while an athlete with a high absolute strength would be more successful in accelerating external objects such as a shotput or ball. Achieving maximum acceleration depends upon the development of large forces at both low and high velocities; to this end there is an advantage to possessing a high proportion of fast twitch muscle fibers in the appropriate muscles, as discussed above in the section *Factors Affecting Strength Performance.*

PURPOSES OF TESTING STRENGTH AND POWER

Four purposes of testing strength and power are presented below. Perhaps the two most common purposes are (2) and (3). Consultation among the sport scientists, the coaches, and the athletes is normally used to establish the purposes of the testing.

1. Determining the Relevance and Relative Importance of Strength and Power to Performance

There may be a few sports in which the relevance of strength and power is uncertain. There may be many sports in which the relevance of strength and power is certain, but their relative importance is uncertain. In sports where both relevance and relative importance of strength and power are certain, there may be uncertainty about the best training program design. It may be possible to resolve all of these uncertainties by appropriate testing of strength and power.

By correlating the results of specific tests of strength and power with sport performance, the relevance and relative importance of strength and power to performance can be established. An example of this process was presented above in the section *RELEVANCE AND RELATIVE IMPORTANCE OF STRENGTH AND POWER TO SPORT PERFORMANCE.* The process is most easily applied to "strength-endurance" sports involving a single "closed" skill (e.g., rowing, swimming, running, flat-water canoeing). The process is more

difficult and complicated in sports which involve several skill patterns which are "open" (i.e., performance influenced by tactics, response to opponent's actions, etc.). Examples of these sports are tennis, volleyball, and downhill skiing. The process can be simplified somewhat in these sports by correlating tests of strength and power with single measurable skills (e.g., velocity of tennis serve, velocity of volleyball spike), rather than overall performance.

If this process were conducted successfully, the coach would acquire information that would allow him/her to establish the priority that should be placed upon training for strength and power. In addition, information may be produced which aids in the design of the training program (e.g., movement patterns to be emphasized, velocity of the training).

It is important to emphasize that the success of the process and the validity of the conclusions formed will depend critically upon the degree to which the tests of strength and power have been specific. The administration of irrelevant, nonspecific tests could result in the formulation of erroneous conclusions; the subsequent action taken could have a serious effect on the progress of the athletes.

2. Development of an Athlete Profile

Most sports require several qualities for successful performance: strength and power, aerobic and anaerobic power, flexibility, skill, and judgment. Within a sport, elite athletes will have strengths and weaknesses in relation to these qualities. A battery of appropriate, specific tests of these qualities administered to a group of athletes would allow a profile of each athlete to be made. With such a profile in hand, a coach would be able to modify the overall program for an athlete and to concentrate on improving the weak qualities while maintaining, and if possible improving, the strong qualities.

3. Monitoring Training Progress

The success of strength and power training programs can be evaluated by the administration of tests before and after training periods. Appropriate alterations can be made to the programs based upon the results of the testing.

The monitoring of the progress made in the training itself is often built into the training program. Thus, in weight training, still the most common method of strength training, progress is monitored readily by recording the increases in the weights used for a given range of repetitions. Complementary lab tests of strength may provide additional useful information about training progress; for example, whether strength has increased most at a particular velocity or point in a range of movement. It must be recognized, however, that the most sensitive monitoring of training progress occurs when the same mode (equipment, movement patterns) is used for both training and testing (Thorstensson et al., 1976; Lindh, 1979). Therefore, the lab tests often will not indicate the degree of progress revealed by the built-in tests of the training program. This problem could be solved only by having the athletes train on the lab equipment, a solution which is impractical in almost all cases. The problem of lab tests being insensitive to training progress can be minimized by having the training mode and the testing mode as specific as possible to the sport movement.

Of even greater importance to the coach and athlete is the degree to which the progress in the training enhances performance. The extent of the transfer to performance will vary according to the relevance and relative importance of strength and power to performance, and the degree to which the training has been specific. A gymnast who performs isometric strength training to increase "iron cross" performance on the rings can expect "one to one" transfer from training to performance, while a swimmer performing a specific strength training program might expect only a 1% improvement in sprint performance for every 5% increase in strength as measured on the training apparatus (Sharp et al., 1982).

The quantitation and evaluation of the transfer from training to performance is complicated in sports which require several qualities for success; in particular, when training has been conducted for all of these qualities. By correlating changes in the qualities with the changes in performance, the sport scientist may be able to apportion responsibility for performance improvement or deterioration.

It is important for athletes and coaches to recognize that there may be a wide range in the response to the same training program. For example, a group of seven female track and field athletes performed a strength training program for six months. The average increase in strength was about 35%, but the range was 15 to 53% (Brown and Wilmore, 1974). Several factors could account for this range in improvement, including initial state of training, "talent" for improvement, general state of health, and effort expended by the athletes. It is an oversimplification, although perhaps an attractive one for coaches, to assume that motivation and dedication are the only factors which affect training progress. Unfortunately, it is usually difficult to apportion relative responsibility to the various factors.

4. Monitoring Rehabilitation of Injuries

Athletes may sustain injuries, the recovery from which will require a period of relative inactivity or even immobilization. If pre-injury strength and power data are available for an athlete, the extent of the decrease in strength resulting from the injury can be quantified, as can the course of rehabilitation. When the pre-injury strength and power levels have been reattained or exceeded, recovery can be judged as complete.

METHODS OF MEASURING STRENGTH AND POWER

In this section, the three most common methods of measuring strength and power will be described briefly, followed by a comparison of the methods.

Methods

Weight Lifting

In weight lifting, strength usually is measured as the heaviest weight that can be lifted once (one repetition maximum or 1 RM) through a range of movement. The units of measurement are the newton (N) for weight or kilogram (kg) for mass. The apparatus used for weight lifting tests may consist of "free" weights (barbells and dumbbells) or weight lifting machines (either "off the shelf" machines or those specifically constructed for testing). Calisthenics are a form of weight lifting. A test consists of counting the number of repetitions that can be performed; it is assumed that stronger individuals (i.e., those with higher strength/body mass ratio) can perform more repetitions.

Isometric Testing

In isometric tests, strength is measured as the

peak force or torque developed during a maximal voluntary contraction. The apparatus consists of an isometric dynamometer and a read-out device. The units of measurement are the newton (N) for force or the newton meter (N·m) for torque. Isometric dynamometers are commercially available; in many cases, however, the sport scientist will have to construct a dynamometer that will allow specific sport movement testing and a recording system that will allow a more detailed analysis (e.g., rate of force development).

Isokinetic Testing

The term "isokinetic" means constant velocity (Perrine, 1968). An isokinetic dynamometer allows voluntary contractions to be made at various constant velocities. In theory, once a velocity has been set, it remains constant despite any variation in the magnitude of the torque applied to the dynamometer. An isometric contraction is a special case of isokinetic contraction (constant velocity = 0), but the term "isokinetic" is rarely applied to isometric contractions; rather, it is applied to constant velocity concentric or eccentric contractions. Almost all isokinetic strength testing involves concentric contractions. The well known "Cybex" (Lumex, Inc., Ronkonkoma, New York) is the only commercially available isokinetic dynamometer. The Cybex allows isometric and concentric contraction strength to be measured; strength usually is measured as torque (N·m).

Comparison of Methods

Reliability and Validity

The reliability or reproducibility of measurement is similar for all three methods, with an average test-to-test variation of about 10% (Tornvall, 1963; Thorstensson, 1976). The validity of measurements of strength and power depends more upon the degree to which the tests are specific to the sport movement rather than upon the method of testing *per se*; for a given sport, however, one method may allow specificity to be applied more easily than the others. The isometric method is at a disadvantage in this respect because most sport movements are dynamic rather than static.

Measurement of Strength

In the isometric and isokinetic methods, force or torque is measured directly. In the weight lifting method, it usually is assumed that the force applied to the apparatus is equal to the weight lifted; in fact, the force applied must initially exceed the weight in order to accelerate it from rest. Toward the end of the range of movement, the applied force will be less than the weight as negative acceleration occurs. The weight lifting apparatus could be instrumented to allow the applied force to be measured directly. In tests using calisthenics, strength is predicted on the basis of the number of repetitions performed (Berger, 1967); strength is not measured directly.

The resistance offered by the Cybex (isokinetic dynamometer) through a range of movement matches precisely the strength curve for the movement; therefore, maximal strength through a range of movement can be measured readily and quickly (Figure 3.5). To obtain a similar result in isometric testing, contractions would have to be performed at many joint angles, a process that would be time consuming and fatiguing. In a weight lifting test, the resistance offered by the weight may not vary in accordance with the

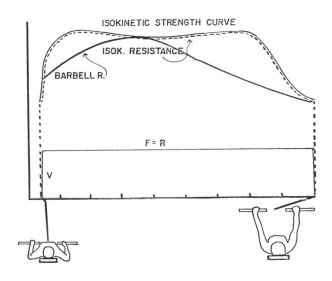

Fig. 3.5 Comparison between a barbell and an isokinetic device in the resistance offered during the bench press exercise. Top solid line shows the strength curve obtained when a maximal contraction was performed at a slow velocity on the isokinetic device. Obviously, the resistance offered by the device (dotted line) precisely matches the strength curve. In contrast, the resistance offered by a barbell does not precisely match the strength curve. Bottom solid line indicates that the velocity (v) of movement was constant (applied force, F, equalled resistance, R) through most of the movement.

strength curve for a movement; therefore, maximal strength may be measured at only one point in the strength curve (Figure 3.5). Some weight lifting machines are designed to provide matching variable resistance; they cannot, however, provide the precision offered by an isokinetic dynamometer because they possess a fixed average resistance curve which cannot adjust for individual variations.

Isometric dynamometers, by definition, can be used to measure only isometric contraction strength. The Cybex is commonly used to measure isometric and concentric contraction strength. The Cybex can be adapted to measure eccentric contraction strength (Rodgers and Berger, 1974) but the adaptation is crude; further, its application is limited by the torque capacity of the Cybex (approximately 500 N·m), unless a gear system is employed. Noncommercial eccentric contraction dynamometers have been constructed for research (e.g., Komi, 1973), and could conceivably be adapted for athlete testing. Eccentric dynamometers are potentially quite dangerous and their design should include robust and reliable safety features. Weight lifting exercise involves alternating concentric and eccentric contraction phases. In a weight lifting test, it is the concentric phase which is tested (i.e., raising the weight). Eccentric weight lifting tests have obvious limitations, one being the determination of a criterion velocity.

In relation to specificity, the limitation of isometric testing for dynamic sport movements has been mentioned. Weight lifting apparatus can be designed to simulate many sport movements. The Cybex is designed to test single joint, unilateral (one limb at a time) movements. The Cybex must be adapted to permit testing of large muscle group, multijoint, bilateral movements. As examples, the Cybex has been adapted to measure bilateral leg press strength (Vandervoort et al., 1981), rowing strength (Pyke et al., 1979) and the torque developed during cycling (Katch et al., 1974). The adaptation for multijoint, bilateral movements must include a gear system which increases the torque capacity of the dynamometer.

Measurement of Power

Power can be determined in the isokinetic method simply by multiplying the force or torque developed by the velocity at which the contraction was made ($P = F \times V$). In the weight lifting method, power can be calculated if the apparatus has been instrumented with a displacement potentiometer or accelerometer. In the isokinetic method, the velocity is controlled, and the power will vary in correspondence to the torque or force generated. In the weight lifting method, the load is controlled, and power will vary in correspondence to the product of the force applied and peak or average velocity attained. The isokinetic system is perhaps a simpler and neater system than the weight lifting system. Power cannot be measured in the isometric method because the velocity is zero.

Force-Velocity Relation

If the strength and power testing is to be specific in relation to contraction velocity, the test method must allow strength to be measured at a wide range of velocities. The Cybex has a velocity range of 0 to 300°/s (0-5.24 rad/s). The upper limit of this range can be extended by a gear system (Vandervoort et al., 1981). Such an extension may be necessary because a velocity of 5.24 rad/s may be less than 50% of maximum velocity for some movements (Thorstensson, 1976). In the weight lifting method, a range of contraction velocities can be achieved by varying the absolute or relative (% 1 RM or % body weight) load against which maximal contractions are made. The relative appropriateness of the isokinetic and weight lifting methods for high velocity strength and power measurements depends upon the nature of the sport movement. In movements where a large mass must be accelerated at the start of a movement, the weight lifting method may be more specific, whereas the isokinetic method may be more suitable when the resistance is met after the limbs or body mass have been accelerated to a high velocity (Figure 3.6). Jumping and throwing are examples of the former case while kicking a ball, the slap shot in hockey, and the volleyball spike are examples of the latter case.

Isometric strength can, of course, be measured at only one velocity. High velocity strength performance may possibly be inferred, however, from the measurement of rate of force development of isometric contractions.

Fatigue Tests

The methods which have been described are used most often to measure the strength and pow-

HIGH SPEED TRAINING

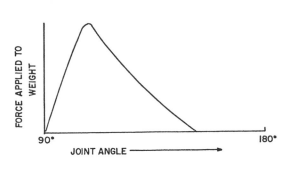

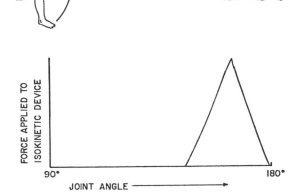

Fig. 3.6 High velocity training with weights and an isokinetic device. Top: The graph shows the force applied to a weight in knee extension with a ballistic action. Great force must be applied initially to accelerate the weight. By the time a high velocity has been attained at the end of the movement, the applied force will have declined greatly or even ceased. Bottom: In performing high velocity contractions on an isokinetic device, the trainee must first accelerate the limb to attain and attempt to exceed the velocity of the device before it will offer resistance to movement. Thus, the device will offer no resistance (save the inertia of the lever arm) at the beginning of the movement but will offer resistance near the end of the movement.

er of single, maximal contractions. These methods also may be used to administer "fatigue" tests. These tests are used to assess endurance, to determine a fatigue "index", or to measure anaerobic power (see Chapter 5). On the Cybex, a typical fatigue test usually consists of 50 to 100 consecutive maximal contractions performed at moderate velocity (e.g., π rad/s); a fatigue index is calculated as the decline in torque during the test (Thorstensson and Karlsson, 1976). In weight lift-

ing, a test of endurance might consist of performing as many repetitions as possible with a particular absolute or relative load. In the isometric method, a fatigue index may be obtained if a maximal contraction is sustained for 1 to 2 min; alternatively, an endurance test might consist of maintaining a given absolute or relative force (% MVC) as long as possible. Significant correlations between fatigability and muscle fiber composition have been demonstrated in both isokinetic (Thorstensson and Karlsson, 1976) and isometric exercise (Hulten et al., 1975); presumably, a similar correlation would be found in weight lifting. As in the case of strength and power measurements, fatigue tests should be as sport specific as possible.

RECOMMENDED PROCEDURES

Weight Lifting

Equipment

The equipment should allow the test to be specific with respect to the sport movement pattern. In the case of some fortunate sports, specific weight lifting equipment may be available commercially; in many sports, however, modification of commercially available equipment will be necessary. In some cases, specific apparatus will have to be constructed. The design of the equipment should also allow the athlete to make maximal contractions comfortably and safely; the former is achieved by appropriate padding and upholstery, and the latter is achieved by strategically placed safety stops, which will prevent an athlete from being crushed or otherwise injured by a heavy weight. If free weights (barbells) are to be used for testing, power racks can provide the element of safety.

Calibration

It is a good practice to be skeptical of the weight values stamped on free weight plates or the plates of machine weight stacks. An independent weighing with an accurate weigh scale, at the point of force application, with subsequent relabelling if necessary, is recommended. In the case of free weight plates, the machined "Olympic" plates are usually closer to the stated weight than the cheaper cast plates.

Measurement of Strength

1 RM

The one repetition maximum (1 RM), that is, the heaviest weight that can be lifted once, is the most common measure of weight lifting strength (Figure 3.7). Although repetitions in weight lifting involve alternating concentric and eccentric contraction phases (Figure 3.7), a weight lifting test almost always is a test of concentric contraction strength.

Positioning

It is important to standardize the starting position and range of movement of the test movements. Standardization reduces to a minimum un-

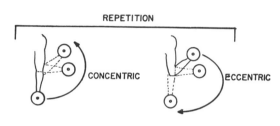

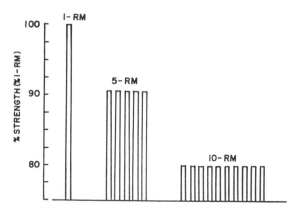

Fig. 3.7 The Repetition Maximum. Top: In weight lifting exercise, the term "repetition" refers to one execution of an exercise movement. A repetition usually consists of a concentric and an eccentric contraction phase. In weight lifting strength tests, it is the concentric contraction strength that is measured. The "repetition maximum" (RM) is the greatest weight than can be used for a designated number of repetitions. Bottom: The 1 RM by definition requires 100% of 1 RM strength. The weight used for the 5 and 10 RM would correspond to a lesser percentage of the 1 RM, as illustrated.

wanted variability in the test results. For example, variation in a starting position which occurs on the steep portion of a strength curve would cause a marked variation in the results. Standardization usually is achieved by designating specific joint angles as the starting position. The actual joint angles selected would, of course, depend on the sport movement pattern.

The force of a concentric contraction can be enhanced by preceding it with an eccentric contraction of the same muscle group. This "rebound effect" would introduce a complicating variability to the results of weight lifting tests. Consequently, it is a good practice to eliminate the rebound effect from the test by having the test consist of an isolated concentric contraction.

Number of trials

Unlike isometric or isokinetic testing, in which two or three maximal contractions can be requested following a few submaximal warm-up contractions, the 1 RM must be "hunted for" with a series of one repetition sets with increasingly heavier weights. It is important that the lead-up sets be not too numerous, or fatigue will affect the final result; in addition, a rest period of 2 to 3 min between successive trials will help to minimize the development of fatigue. As the athlete and the tester gain experience with the 1 RM protocol, the number of lead-up sets will become optimal, that is, a sufficient number for adequate warm-up but not so many as to cause fatigue.

Instructions to subjects

Performance on a weight lifting test is optimal when an effort is made to contract as hard and as fast as possible, and subjects should be instructed accordingly. Standardization of these instructions and the degree of encouragement offered will help to minimize variation in the test results.

Measurement of Power

Instrumentation

In order to obtain a measure of power in weight lifting, a means of measuring velocity of movement must be incorporated into the test apparatus. Perhaps the simplest approach would be to mount a displacement potentiometer onto the apparatus. This would allow average velocity attained during the test movement to be determined, which, multiplied by the weight of the mass lifted, would provide a value for power. Of course, the true power value would be obtained by multiplying the average velocity by the actual average force developed during the lift. The actual force could be measured by instrumenting the apparatus with strain gauges or an accelerometer.

Protocols

Several protocols for measuring power are possible. The simplest procedure would be to multiply the 1 RM by the average velocity attained during the lift or, if force has been measured directly, by multiplying the average force by the average velocity. In practice, however, the variation in velocity of 1 RM executions would be small; aside from being able to express the test results in units of power, little further information would be gained. More productive approaches could be used. Force and/or average velocity could be measured with various absolute or relative (% 1 RM) weights; thus, a force- and power-velocity relationship could be determined. The focus of the analysis could be directed upon the range of velocities relevant to the sport performance. (The relative merits of isokinetic and weight lifting tests in relation to high velocity strength and power measurement have been discussed above, p. 16).

Positioning

As in the case of the 1 RM test, standardization of the starting position and range of movement is important. The test movement should consist of an isolated concentric contraction in order to avoid the variability that would be caused by the rebound effect. It could be argued that this principle should be violated if the sport movement involves the rebound effect. The argument is a good one; great care must be taken, however, to ensure that the equipment provides the necessary safety features. The challenge would be to design the apparatus to allow unrestricted application of the rebound effect while at the same time including safety stops to prevent injury.

Number of trials

Following a few warm-up trials, the recommended procedure would be to have the subject perform 2 to 3 maximal efforts at each load.

Instructions

It is important that subjects understand that contractions should be as forceful and rapid as possible. Terms like "accelerate" and "explode" may help to get the message across.

Fatigue Tests

Relative and absolute loads

In weight lifting, fatigue tests consist of performing as many repetitions as possible with a designated absolute or relative (% 1 RM) load. If the sport involves supporting the body weight, the designated load may be a percentage of body weight. Determination of the optimum load to use may require preliminary experimentation. For example, it may be desirable that the load selected for a fatigue test for rowers be one which causes fatigue (i.e., inability to continue performing repetitions) within 4 to 7 min, a duration corresponding approximately to the duration of the rowing race. In rowing, it is probably most appropriate to determine, by experimentation, an absolute load (e.g., a power output which, if sustained over 2000 m, would "smash" the current world record) which would cause fatigue within the specified time range.

It has already been pointed out (p. 12) that while a positive correlation exists between strength and absolute endurance (the ability to sustain a high absolute force or power), a negative correlation exists between strength and relative endurance (the ability to sustain a given percentage of maximum strength or power). Thus, a relatively strong or powerful athlete may have a relatively high absolute endurance; this athlete, however, will have a relatively low relative endurance if the high strength performance is due to a genetically endowed high proportion of fast twitch muscle fibers in the involved muscles, or to strength training, which increases the percent fast twitch fiber area within the muscles. Therefore, in this athlete (and in most athletes) relative and absolute endurance tests would lead to opposite conclusions about the endurance capacity of the athlete. It is clear, then, that the appropriate choice of a fatigue test (absolute vs. relative) for a given sport is critical.

Repetition rate

The time taken to perform each repetition with a

weight and the duration of the intervals between the repetitions will affect the number of repetitions that can be performed. This source of variation can be eliminated by having the repetitions performed at a standardized rate. Standardization can be achieved by use of a metronome set to the appropriate frequency.

Rebound effect

Variation in the degree to which the rebound effect is employed in performing repetitions will have a marked effect on the outcome of fatigue tests. It is therefore important to standardize the degree to which the rebound effect is utilized. In practice, the simplest approach is to attempt to eliminate the rebound effect entirely. This can be done by introducing a pronounced pause between the eccentric and concentric phases of each repetition. The pause can be reinforced by equipment design; a stop can be provided on which the weight rests during the pauses. The pause and momentary unloading of the muscle allow the rebound effect to be dissipated.

Isometric Tests

Equipment

In most cases a frame will have to be constructed to permit testing of the sport specific movement pattern (e.g., Secher, 1975). The frame would then be instrumented appropriately with a commercially available force transducer (load cell) or with strain gauges. The read-out device could be an oscilloscope or good quality pen recorder. A three-channel recorder would be convenient, for it would allow simultaneous recording of force, rate of force development, and the force-time integral (Figure 3.8). Of course, an alternative would be computer analysis of the input signal from the transducer, with subsequent print-out and graphic display of the desired measurements. (The same approach to recording and computer analysis also could be applied to the weight lifting method in relation to the measurement of displacement, velocity, force, and power; see above).

Calibration

Isometric dynamometers are calibrated with known weights. It is important that calibration is done throughout the working range of the instru-

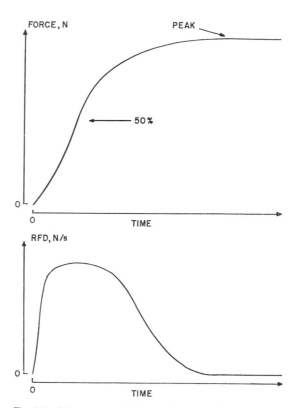

Fig. 3.8 Measurement of isometric strength and rate of force development (RFD). Top: With suitable instrumentation (see text), a force-time curve can be obtained from maximal isometric contractions. Peak force is readily obtained. Average RFD up to any point (e.g., 50% of peak force) on the force-time curve can be calculated by dividing the force obtained by the time taken to attain that point. Bottom: Alternatively, the first differential of the force-time signal could be displayed on a second channel, from which the peak RFD could be directly read.

ment. Frequent calibration over a period of time will establish the stability of the system and indicate the frequency at which calibration should be done. It may be prudent to calibrate before each testing session, particularly when considerable time elapses between sessions.

Measurement of Strength

Peak force or torque

Strength is measured as the peak force (newtons, N) or torque (newton meters, N·m) developed during a maximal voluntary contraction (Figure 3.8).

Positioning

It is important that body positioning (joint angles) be standardized. Variation in positioning which occurs on the steep portion of a strength curve would cause a marked variation in the results (Figure 3.9). Even when the test is for a single joint only, it still may be necessary to standardize other joint angles. For example, the isometric force developed in knee extension is affected by variation in the hip joint angle (Currier, 1977), presumably by varying the length of the rectus femoris.

Number of trials

Following a few submaximal warm-up contractions, a test consists of 2 to 3 brief maximal contractions with rest periods of about one minute between successive contractions. The best performance or the average of the best two trials can be taken as the measure of performance, although reproducibility of the measurement apparently is not improved by taking the average of trials rather than the best trial (Alderman and Banfield, 1969).

Instructions to subjects

Performance in isometric strength tests can be influenced by the instructions which are given on how to perform the contractions (Kroemer and Howard, 1970). Thus, instructing a subject to "jerk" will produce a different result than "raise slowly to a maximum and hold." Therefore, instructions to subjects should be standardized. When it is intended to measure rate of force development as well as peak force, the appropriate instruction would be: "Contract as hard and as fast as possible!" The contractions need last only a few seconds.

Measurement of Rate of Force Development

Rate of force development (RFD) is a measure of the time rate at which force or torque is developed; the units are newtons per second ($N \cdot s^{-1}$) and newton meters per second ($N \cdot m \cdot s^{-1}$), respectively. One approach to measuring RFD is illustrated in Figure 3.8. The peak force simply is divided by the time taken to reach peak force. There are two problems with this approach. First, it is difficult to determine when the peak force is first attained because of the shape of the force-time curve (Figure 3.8). Second, the contractions may not always be as smooth as shown in Figure 3.8 as the peak is approached; there may be dips and bumps in the force-time record which would cause large variations in the time to peak force. These two problems can be obviated by selecting a point on the smooth portion of the force-time curve which represents a particular percentage (e.g., 50%) of the peak force attained (Figure 3.8). RFD would be measured as the force representing the selected percentage of peak force divided by the time elapsed in attaining the selected percentage of peak force. The selection of a percentage of peak force is arbitrary. It can be seen in Figure 3.8 that the calculated value for RFD will vary depending on the percentage of peak force that is selected, but this variation does not present a problem provided that the same percentage always is used for calculation.

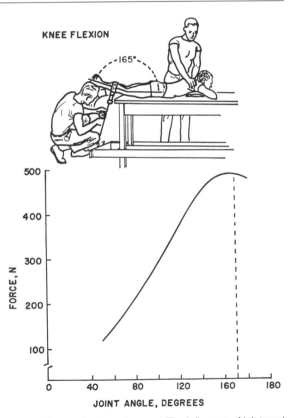

Fig. 3.9 Isometric strength curve. The influence of joint position on the isometric strength of the knee flexors is illustrated. The marked variation in force with changing joint angle serves to emphasize the importance of standardizing joint angles in isometric strength measurement. Redrawn from Clarke (1966).

The quickest and most convenient method for measuring RFD is to have the first differential of the force-time event determined electronically (Figure 3.8). A suitable recorder would allow RFD (first differential) to be displayed below the force-time record (Figure 3.8). The peak rate of force development can be read off the recording. Alternatively, appropriate computer analysis of the force-time signal would produce a print-out and graphic diplay of the peak RFD.

The guidelines related to positioning, number of trials, and instructions are the same as those presented above for measuring peak force. In particular, subjects should be instructed to contract as hard and as fast as possible.

Fatigue Tests

In the isometric condition, a fatigue test may consist of maintaining a given relative or absolute force as long as possible, or maintaining a maximal voluntary contraction for a specified time period, with subsequent calculation of a fatigue index (Figure 3.10).

Relative vs. absolute loads

An isometric fatigue (endurance) test may consist of sustaining a particular percentage of maximum strength (relative load) as long as possible. A second type of relative loading would be to designate the force to be sustained as a percentage of body weight. Alternatively, the test may consist of sustaining a given absolute force as long as possible. The choice of test will depend upon the nature of the sport. For example, for downhill skiing, an appropriate test may be sustaining a given percentage (e.g., 150%) of body weight as long as possible.

The relationship between strength and endurance has been discussed above (p. 12 and 19), namely, that there is a positive correlation between strength and absolute endurance but a negative correlation between strength and relative endurance. Thus, in the case of an athlete with a high level of strength, absolute and relative fatigue or endurance tests could lead easily to opposite conclusions about the endurance capacity of the athlete. In the downhill skiing example, an athlete with a high strength/body weight ratio would fare well on a fatigue test based on sustaining a given percentage of body weight, but would perform relatively poorly on a fatigue test based on a

percentage of absolute strength; the former test would be the appropriate one for skiing. It is clear, therefore, that careful consideration must be given to selecting the fatigue test which is most relevant to the sport performance.

Fatigue index vs. force-time integral and average force

Rather than sustaining a given absolute or relative force as long as possible, a fatigue test could consist of maintaining a maximal voluntary con-

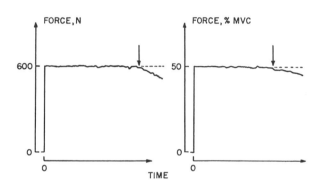

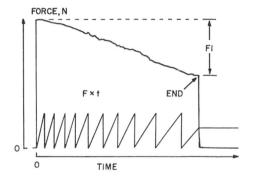

Fig. 3.10.   Isometric fatigue tests. Top left: The test consists of maintaining a given absolute force as long as possible (usually submaximal). Top right: The test consists of maintaining a given relative (e.g., 50% MVC) force as long as possible. Bottom: In the test an MVC is performed and maximal effort is maintained for a designated time period (e.g., 1.0 min) despite the decline in force. A fatigue index (FI) can be calculated as the % decline in force during the test. A second channel could record the integration of force and time (F × t); the saw-tooth wave form illustrates one type of display of the integration. Thus, the upper peak of each "tooth" would indicate "x" N·s. The average force developed during the test could be calculated as the total integration divided by the elapsed time. The relative merits of these fatigue tests are discussed in the text.

traction for a specified time period (Figure 3.10). A fatigue index could be calculated as the percent decline in force over the time period. In addition, integration of the force-time event would allow the force-time integral (in N·s) and average force to be determined (Figure 3.10): these latter measurements may be more useful than the fatigue index. For example, a paddler may have a greater percent decline in power in a race than another paddler; nevertheless, the first paddler will still have the better performance if his/her average power over the race was greater. This point will be discussed in more detail below in connection with isokinetic testing (p. 29).

Administration of fatigue tests

When the test consists of maintaining a particular absolute or relative force as long as possible, a method for displaying the required force level to the subject must be present. Examples would be beam matching on an oscilloscope, or maintaining a given value on a digital read-out device. In practice, the force level may fluctuate plus or minus a few percent of the required force early in the test, and later the percent fluctuation may increase. It is therefore necessary to impress upon the subjects the importance of keeping the force as steady as possible. It falls to the administrator to establish the criterion for ending the test.

By comparison, it is perhaps easier to administer the sustained MVC type of test. The subject contracts as strongly as possible for the specified time period. The administrator should emphasize to the subject the importance of making and keeping the effort maximal throughout the test; there should be no pacing.

Fatigue tests will be associated with discomfort in the fatiguing muscles; in fact, mental toughness will be a factor affecting performance on fatigue tests. Pain caused by inappropriate padding or body support braces should not, however, be part of the test. The design of the apparatus should ensure comfort in the performance of tests, save the unavoidable discomfort which emanates from the contracting muscles.

Isokinetic Tests

Equipment

Currently (1982), there is only one commercially available isokinetic dynamometer, the well-known Cybex (Lumex, Inc., Ronkonkoma, New York). "Home-made" isokinetic dynamometers have been constructed for laboratory research (e.g., Komi, 1973). The construction features of the Cybex dynamometer have not been published, but the dynamometer apparently consists of a small DC servomotor employing tachometer feedback control. Once a particular velocity has been set, the motor resists acceleration that would otherwise be caused by applied torques. Thus, the isokinetic (constant velocity) condition has been achieved. In practice, the application of large torques, particularly at the higher velocities, will cause a brief acceleration of the servomotor before "settling down" to the preset velocity (Thorstensson et al., 1976). In the construction of a home-made dynamometer, this acceleration could be reduced or eliminated by using a more powerful motor.

The Cybex allows torque to be applied and measured in two opposite directions; that is, the shaft of the dynamometer can rotate clockwise and anti-clockwise. Certainly, the servomotor doesn't rotate in both directions; hence the bi-directional capability is probably achieved by the use of a pair of unidirectional gears.

A notable safety feature of the Cybex is that the shaft does not rotate with the motor. The shaft must be accelerated (by the subject) and will engage the servomotor when its velocity matches that of the motor; in fact, engagement occurs when the subject attempts to accelerate the shaft beyond the preset velocity of the servomotor. The principle underlying this feature may be similar to that used on a bicycle (the wheel being analogous to the rotating servomotor and the chain and sprocket assembly being analogous to the shaft). It would be prudent to include this feature in any home-made isokinetic device.

Torque capacity

Usually torque rather than force is measured on the Cybex. The construction of the Cybex (rotating shaft) lends itself to measuring the strength of single joint movements; the axis of the joint selected is aligned with the axis of the Cybex shaft. With this arrangement, measuring torque rather than force is more appropriate and convenient (Figure 3.11).

The manufacturer of the Cybex rates the torque capacity of the Cybex as 360 ft·lb (488 N·m). This capacity is sufficient for measuring the strength of

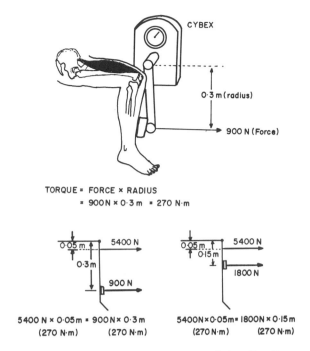

Fig. 3.11.   Measurement of torque on the Cybex. Top: Torque is equal to the force applied to the shin pad multiplied by the radius (distance between axis of dynamometer and shin pad; note that axis of knee joint is aligned with axis of dynamometer). Bottom: The torque measured is the torque developed by the involved muscles (in this example the quadriceps, F = 5400 N, inserted 0.05 m from the joint axis). The shin pad can be placed anywhere on the lower leg; the torque measurement will not vary, although the force applied to the shin pad will vary.

most single joint, unilateral movements. Some very strong athletes may exceed this limit in low velocity knee extension, and even non-athletes may exceed the torque capacity in low velocity hip extension. Off the shelf, the Cybex is not suitable for bilateral, single joint testing; the dynamometer must be coupled to an apparatus constructed for the purpose of bilateral testing. Having achieved that, there remains the problem of the torque capacity of the Cybex. Low and even moderately high velocity bilateral knee extension would surely exceed the capacity of the Cybex. Tests would have to be restricted to relatively small muscle groups (e.g., elbow flexors).

Many sports involve large muscle group, multijoint, bilateral movements. The torques developed in these movements could well exceed 1000 or even 2000 N·m. The question arises as to how the Cybex could be adapted to measure such large torques. The adaptation consists of coupling the Cybex to an apparatus which includes an appropriate gear assembly. The appropriate gear ratio will increase the torque capacity as desired. Such an adaptation has been applied to strength testing of rowers (Pyke et al., 1979) and to the measurement of leg press (involving hip and knee extension) strength (Vandervoort et al., 1981). It should be pointed out that gearing to increase torque capacity reduces the velocity limit; for example, a gear ratio (2:1) which doubles the torque capacity halves the velocity limit. This may be a problem depending on the nature of the sport.

Velocity limit

The velocity limit of the currently marketed Cybex is 300°/s or 50 rpm (5.24 rad·s^{-1}). This velocity represents about 50% of the average velocity of unresisted (save inertia and weight of the lower leg) knee extension (10 rad·s^{-1}, Thorstensson, 1976). Similar average velocities probably are attained at the elbow joint. The velocity limit of the Cybex can be increased by a gear system; it is achieved, however, at the expense of torque capacity. For example, a gear ratio which doubles the velocity limit halves the torque capacity. At first, this may not seem to be a problem because the torque of maximal concentric contractions decreases as velocity increases. Our experience with large muscle group, multijoint, bilateral movements (leg press and bench press), however, has indicated that the decline in torque capacity with gearing into the mid-velocity range exceeds the decline in the *in vivo* torque-velocity relation. Thus, caution should be exercised when a protocol is being developed which involves gearing to increase the velocity limit; a lack of caution could result in damage to the Cybex servomotor. In the construction of a home-made isokinetic dynamometer, a greater torque and velocity limit can be achieved by using a more powerful servomotor.

Read-out device

Currently, the Cybex package includes a two-channel thermal recorder; one channel displays torque and the second channel displays angular displacement. A three-channel recorder would be an improvement, for it would allow the integration of torque and time to be displayed. The torque-time integral allows average torque and power and work to be determined easily (see below and

Figure 3.12). Better still, the signal from the transducer could be fed into a computer, with a subsequent print-out and/or graphic display of the desired measurements. The makers of Cybex have recently introduced a computerized analysis package.

Calibration

Torque

The manufacturer of the Cybex provides an attachment for calibration of torque. Known weights are placed on the attachment, which is positioned above the horizontal plane. The attachment is then released and the peak torque is registered as the attachment passes through the horizontal plane. This type of calibration is feasible at low velocities only, but it has been assumed that the calibration would be applicable to the whole velocity range. Recently, however, it has been demonstrated that different torque calibrations are required for different velocity settings (Olds et al., 1981; Murray et al., 1982). This may be a troublesome characteristic of the pressure transducer which is part of the Cybex. The effect is considerable; for example, Olds et al. (1981) found the calibration factor for a statically applied load to be 5.38 V/N·m but at 180°/s (π rad $\times$ s^{-1}) the factor was 6.37 V/N·m, an 18.4% increase. The prospect of calibrating at all test velocities is dismaying; perhaps the better course of action would be to forego the Cybex pressure transducer entirely and mount a torque strain transducer (commercially available) on the Cybex shaft. This type of transducer is specifically designed to measure torques accurately regardless of variation in angular velocity. The existence of such transducers should be borne in mind when constructing home-made isokinetic dynamometers.

Calibration should include applying known torques throughout the working range of the dynamometer. For further details on calibration, see the section on isometric testing (p. 20).

Velocity

The manufacturer of the Cybex recommends that velocity settings be calibrated by rotating the shaft (engaged with the servomotor) for a given time period (e.g., 1.0 min) and counting the revolutions, or, alternatively, timing the performance of a given number of revolutions. A second approach would be to use the displacement potentiometer to verify velocity settings. Similar procedures could be applied to home-made dynamometers.

Measurement of Strength

Peak torque

Strength usually is measured on the Cybex as the peak torque (units: N·m) developed during a maximal concentric contraction. In some situations, it may be preferable to take as the measurement the torque developed at a particular point in the range of movement.

A phenomenon unique (cf. weight lifting and isometric testing) to concentric contractions performed on an isokinetic dynamometer is the "impact artifact" which occurs when the accelerating limb catches up to the velocity of the servomotor and engages it. The impact artifact had been noted by Thorstensson et al. (1976) and Perrine and Edgerton (1979) and has been dealt with in more detail recently by Winter et al. (1981), Murray et al. (1982), and Sapega et al. (1982). The impact artifact is brought about as the momentum of the accelerating limb is absorbed by the servomotor; that is, the servomotor decelerates the limb, and the torque required to decelerate the limb is recorded as a peak at the beginning of the torque-time recording. The artifact can be present at all velocities but is most pronounced at high velocities (Figure 3.13) because greater momentum has been developed within the moving parts (limb, attachments) at the moment when the servomotor is engaged. This, together with the fact that the torque capacity of the involved muscles is reduced at high constant velocity causes the ratio of the impact artifact torque value to the average torque of the whole event to be much greater for high than for low velocity contractions (Figure 3.13).

The question arises as to whether the impact artifact should be used as the measurement of strength when it represents the peak torque developed during the contraction, as it often will at high velocities. If the purpose of the test is to determine the peak of a strength curve caused by the interaction of the length-tension effect and varying muscle angle of pull (see p. 8), then the impact artifact should be ignored. It also can be argued that the artifact reflects the momentum of the limb and attachments almost entirely and would be present even if the muscles were relaxed at the time of its occurrence. On the other hand,

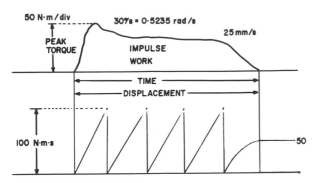

PEAK TORQUE = 50 N·m/div × 5 div = 250 N·m
IMPULSE = 450 N·m·s
TIME = 75 mm / 25mm/s = 3·0 s
AVERAGE TORQUE(IMPULSE/TIME) = 450 N·m·s / 3·0 s = 150 N·m
WORK (IMPULSE × VELOCITY) = 450 N·m·s × 0·5235 rad/s = 235·6 J
AVERAGE POWER (WORK/TIME) = 235·6 J / 3·0 s = 78·5 W
PEAK POWER (PEAK TORQUE × VELOCITY) = 250 N·m × 0·5235 rad/s = 130·9 W

WORK = (IMPULSE) × (VELOCITY)
    = (AVERAGE TORQUE × TIME) × (DISPLACEMENT/TIME)
    = 150 N·m × 1·571 rad (90°) = 235·6 J

AVERAGE POWER = (WORK) / TIME
    = (AVERAGE TORQUE × DISPLACEMENT) / TIME
    = AVERAGE TORQUE × VELOCITY
    = 150 N·m × 0·5235 rad/s
    = 78·5 W

Fig. 3.12. Analysis of Cybex recording. One channel of the recorder displays torque; the other channel displays the integration of torque and time (i.e., "impulse"). The commercial Cybex recorder displays angular displacement with the second channel. To measure peak torque, one simply notes the maximal "height" of the recording in paper divisions and multiplies by the amplification setting (in this example 50 N·m/div.). The integrator was calibrated to 100 N·m·s per full sweep. Thus the "impulse" was 4.5 sweeps or 450 N·m·s. Time of the contraction is determined from the paper speed (25 mm/s) and the "length" of the contraction (75 mm) on the paper. Average torque is calculated as impulse divided by time. Peak torque, average torque and impulse can be converted to peak power, average power, and work respectively by multiplying by the angular velocity (0.5235 rad/s) at which the contractions are made. Note that work and average power can be determined in two different ways. The makers of the Cybex have recently marketed a computer analysis system which does all of the above and more.

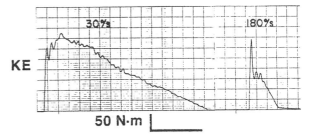

KE

50 N·m

Fig. 3.13 The "impact artifact". The impact artifact (Winter et al., 1981) is illustrated in undamped knee extension recordings. At the lower velocity (left, 30°/s) the impact peak (first peak) is exceeded later in the contraction. At the higher velocity (right, 180°/s) the impact artifact is quite pronounced and is the highest torque level attained during the contraction. See text for the interpretation of the impact artifact.

event which would be considered a troublesome artifact in some contexts (e.g., strength curve determination or true torque-velocity relations) may provide the most valuable information in relation to some sport performances. A compromise would be to use average torque (see below) rather than peak torque as the measure of strength. At low velocities, the impact artifact will have little effect on the value for average torque. At very high velocities, however, the impact artifact may represent most of the recorded event, and the average torque would be the average torque produced by the impact artifact!

Torque-time integral and average torque

Electronic integration and display of the torque-time signal allows the total mechanical effect of the contraction to be measured (Figure 3.12). The units are newton meter seconds (N·m·s). The average torque is obtained simply by dividing the torque time integral by the duration of the contraction (Figure 3.12).

Correction for gravity

In the testing of athletes, consideration is usually given only to the forces or torques developed in excess of those required to support the body or body segment against gravity or to accelerate the mass of the body segments or body as a whole. In the case of strong athletes, these forces or torques will represent only a small percentage of the maximum possible strength. It should be pointed out, however, that when the torques or forces gener-

the magnitude of the artifact does reflect the degree to which the muscles have been able to accelerate the limb prior to engaging the servomotor. In some sport movements (e.g., volleyball spike, kicking), the impact artifact may be the most relevant measurement of all. Again, the guiding principle is specificity in relation to sport performance. It is of interest, however, that a mechanical

ated are relatively small, and a limb must be raised against gravity, the isokinetic dynamometer may only "see" a small portion of the total torque produced. For example, a patient may possess an actual knee extension torque capacity of 50 N·m; 40 N·m are required to raise the lower leg against gravity; the Cybex would record a torque of 10 N·m. In the case of knee flexion assisted by gravity, an actual torque capacity of 20 N·m would be recorded as 60 N·m. By contrast, a strong athlete may develop actual torques of 400 and 200 N.m for knee extension and flexion, respectively. The torque due to gravity would be a relatively small proportion of the total torque developed. If it is determined that correction for gravity is important in strength testing for a particular sport, a method for doing so has been described by Winter et al. (1981). In several sports, a specific strength test would involve movement in a horizontal plane, in which case correction for gravity is not an issue.

Measurement of Power and Work

Power is equal to the product of torque and velocity; thus, the instantaneous power (including the peak power) for any point on a torque-time recording can be obtained by multiplying the torque (N·m) at the point by the angular velocity rad·s^{-1}) used for the test. When the units N·m and rad·s^{-1} (not deg·s^{-1} or rpm) are used for torque and velocity respectively, the proper units of power, namely, watts (W) are obtained (Figure 3.14). Similarly, the average power developed during a contraction may be obtained by multiplying the average torque by the angular velocity (Figures 3.12 and 3.15).

The work done during a contraction can be obtained (Figures 3.12 and 3.15) by multiplying the torque-time integral or "impulse" (N·m·s) by the angular velocity (rad·s^{-1}). Thus:

$$N \cdot m \cdot s \times \left(\frac{m}{m} \times \frac{1}{s} \right) = N \cdot m = J \text{ (joule)}$$

The joule (J) is the SI unit for work and energy.

Selection of Velocity

The selection of velocities for isokinetic testing will depend, of course, on the nature of the sport movement to be tested. It has become conventional to administer tests at the lower and upper limits of the velocity range of the dynamometer (for the Cybex 0-5.24 rad·s^{-1} or 0-300 deg·s^{-1} or

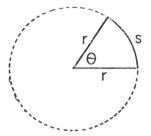

WHEN s = r, θ = 57.307° = 1.0 radians (rad)

360° = 2 π rad (π = 3.141)

IF θ IS IN rad, $\theta = \dfrac{s}{r}$ $\theta(rad) = \dfrac{s(m)}{r(m)}$

WORK = AVERAGE TORQUE × DISPLACEMENT

= N·m × rad   BUT rad = $\dfrac{m}{m}$

= N·m × m/m

= N·m

= J

Fig. 3.14.   Angular displacement. Angular displacement may be expressed in degrees or radians. A radian is the angular displacement when the radius (r) of a circle equals the linear arc(s) of the circle. Because the perimeter (circumference) of a circle = 2πr, then there are 2π rad in a circle. Note that a radian is the ratio of two linear displacements (s/r or m/m). By using radians and radians per second in conjunction with torque, the proper units for work (J) and power (W), respectively, are obtained.

0-50 rpm). Certainly, the velocity considered to be most specific to a sport performance should also be included in the protocol.

The relative merits of high velocity isokinetic and weight lifting tests have been discussed above (p. 16) and should be considered.

In selecting a low velocity for isokinetic measurements, it should be borne in mind that contractions which last longer than a few seconds may be affected by fatigue (Perrine and Edgerton, 1978). This could affect the values of average torque and work produced by test contractions.

Fatigue Tests

The most common fatigue test used with the isokinetic dynamometer is the knee extension fatigue test described by Thorstensson and Karlsson (1976). The test consists of 50 consecutive

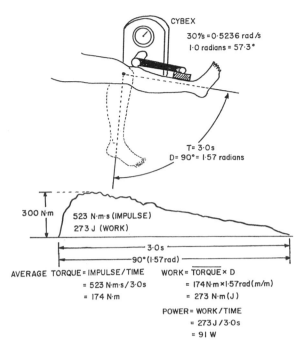

Fig. 3.15. Mechanical properties measured on the Cybex. Top: Knee extension is performed at a velocity of 30°/s through a range of approximately 90°. Middle: A recording of a concentric contraction shows a peak torque of 300 N·m. The torque-time integral ("impulse") was 523 N·m·s. It can be determined by planimetry, electronically or by computer analysis. Bottom: The average torque was calculated as impulse divided by time. Work was calculated as average torque multiplied by displacement, and power was calculated as work divided by time. See also Fig. 3.12.

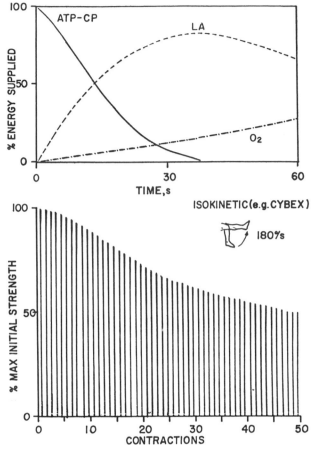

Fig. 3.16. Schematic representation of the common Cybex fatigue test. Bottom: Fifty knee extension contractions were performed at a joint angular velocity of 180°/s. Each contraction lasted about 0.5 s and the time for all 50 contractions was about 1.0 min. The torque declined to about 50% of the initial value during the test; thus, the fatigue index (FI) was 50%. Top: Estimated relative contributions of the three energy systems (LA = lactic acid system) during the course of a test are illustrated. The message is that this test is primarily an anaerobic event.

knee extensions at 3.141 rad·s^{-1} (180 deg·s^{-1}). The percent decline in torque over the 50 contractions is calculated and expressed as a fatigue index. Fifty contractions were found to be optimal; performing an additional 50 contractions caused little further decline in torque and doubled the duration of the test. In a group of ten sedentary men, a positive correlation (r = 0.86) was found between the fatigue index and the percentage of fast twitch fibers within vastus lateralis (Thorstensson and Karlsson, 1976). A schematic representation of this fatigue test is illustrated in Figure 3.16 and the actual results of a test are shown in Figure 3.17.

This basic protocol can be applied to any movement. The selection of velocity is arbitrary. In knee extension, a velocity of 3.141 (π) rad·s^{-1} permitted a 0.5 s contraction phase and a 0.7 s passive recovery phase. A limitation of using low velocities

for fatigue tests on the Cybex is that the dynamometer resists in both directions; thus, a 3 s contraction phase must be followed by a 3 s recovery phase. This work to recovery ratio may delay unduly the fatigue process. This problem could be obviated by mounting a ratchet mechanism on the Cybex shaft. The ratchet would permit a rapid, unresisted recovery phase between the longer work phases, ensuring a rapid rate of fatigue. Fatigue tests involving slow contractions may be most specific for some sports.

50 N·m / div   100 N·m·s / reset

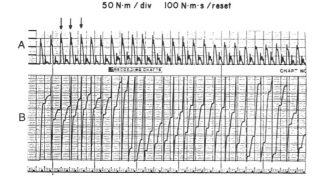

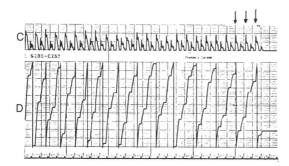

Fig. 3.17.   Recording of Cybex fatigue test. Torque recordings are shown in A and C; the test began at left in A and finished at right in C. The smaller contractions between knee extensions are knee flexions. Subjects usually are instructed to let the leg passively flex between extensions, but many have difficulty complying with this request, particularly as fatigue develops. The fatigue index was calculated on the basis of 3 "early" contractions and the final 3 contractions (see arrows). The initial 3 contractions are not always used because many subjects require a few contractions to build up to their peak value; thus the convention is to take the best 3 of the first 5 or 6 contractions. The fatigue index was 50.6%. The average peak torque over the 50 contractions was 124.5 N·m; therefore, the average peak power was 391 W (124.5 N·m × 3.141 rad/s). To determine the total work output during the test, the impulses of all 50 contractions must be summed (B and D show the channel recording the torque time integral; full sweep = 100 N·m·s). The sum was 2891 N·m·s. The work was 9.1 kJ (2891 N·m·s × 3.141 rad/s).

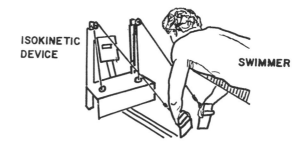

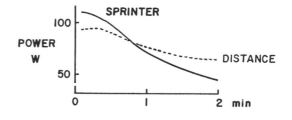

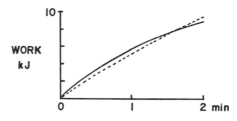

Fig. 3.18.   Fatigability, power and work performance in sprint and distance swimmers. Top: Swimmers performed a fatigue test on a specifically constructed isokinetic "swim bench". Repetitive maximal concentric contractions were performed over a two-minute period. Middle: In the sprinters, the initial power or torque was greater than in the distance swimmers; the sprinters, however, also fatigued more rapidly. Bottom: At one minute, the total work output was greater in the sprinters than in the distance swimmers. By two minutes, the distance swimmers had caught up to and surpassed the sprinters in total work output. Thus, the duration of a work test may greatly affect the conclusions drawn about the work capacity of athletes. See text for further discussion. Redrawn from Thornton and Flavell (1977).

Fatigue index vs. average torque or total work

In addition to calculating the decline in torque or power which occurs in a fatigue test, it is possible, by integration of the torque-time or power-time signal, to calculate the average power and total work output achieved in the test. These latter measurements may be more useful than the fatigue index. In many sports, it is the average power

developed over the duration of the event that is important, rather than the percent decline in power (see Figure 3.18 for an example and Figure 3.17 for sample calculations).

Correction for gravity

Recently, it has been demonstrated that the results of the common knee extension Cybex fatigue test are altered if a correction for gravity is made (Winter et al., 1981). The correlation between corrected and uncorrected (for gravity) fatigue indices in a group of subjects was only $r = 0.80$; no standard error of the estimate was reported. This variation in results should be considered if muscle fiber composition is to be predicted from fatigue test results. In many cases, however, the purpose of fatigue tests for athletes is to determine the average torque or work performed "against" the dynamometer; no "credit" is given for work done in raising a limb against gravity or overcoming the inertia of a limb. In those cases, it could be argued that correction for gravity or inertia is not necessary.

Administration of Tests

Positioning and instructions

The principles of positioning and instructions for isokinetic testing are similar to those for weight lifting tests (p. 18) and isometric tests (p. 21); namely, standardization and consistency. For all methods of strength testing, standardization of positioning can be aided by the use of pads and restraints (straps, etc.) to prevent unwanted variation in positioning. In isokinetic testing, it is important to emphasize to subjects that contractions should be as strong and fast as possible. Words such as "explode", "accelerate", "kick" help to get the message across. In fatigue tests, it is important to emphasize that each contraction be a maximal effort; there should be no pacing.

Number of trials

A few submaximum warm-up contractions followed by 2 to 3 maximal test contractions are usually sufficient for low velocity isokinetic strength measurements. There is more variability in high velocity measurements, and 5 to 6 trials may be needed to obtain good, reproducible results. Thirty- to sixty-second rest intervals seem to be sufficient for low velocity testing, while 10 to 20 s intervals may be sufficient for high velocity testing. Particularly at high velocities, there may be progressive improvement over 3 to 5 successive contractions; this is often observed in fatigue tests (Figure 3.17). This phenomenon serves to emphasize the importance of using at least a few trials, and standardizing the rest periods between trials.

INTERPRETATION OF RESULTS

Units of Measurement

The recommended units for reporting the results of strength and power testing are presented in Table 3.1. The recommended units are the International System of Units (SI).

Units Formed by Multiplication and Division

The product of two or more units in symbolic form should be indicated by a dot (·). The dot preferably should be raised above the line, although it may be on the line if the preferred position is not readily produced.

Example:
N·m for newton meter (not Nm or N-m or N × m)
m·s^{-1} for meters per second (not ms^{-1} or m-s^{-1} or m × s^{-1})

A solidus (oblique stroke /), a horizontal line, or negative powers may be used to express a compound unit formed by division.

Example:
For meters per second: m/s, $\frac{m}{s}$, or m·s^{-1} (not m ÷ s)

Table 3.1   International System of Units (SI) for strength and power measurements.

LINEAR MOTION		ANGULAR MOTION	
Quantity	Unit	Quantity	Unit
Force (F, P, W)	newton (N)	Torque (T)	newton meter (N·m)
Velocity (v)	meters per second (m/s)	Velocity (ω)	radians per second (rad/s)
Mass (m)	kilogram (kg)	Moment of inertia (I, J)	kilogram meter squared (kg·m^2)
Acceleration (a)	meters per second squared (m/s^2)	Acceleration (α)	radians per second squared (rad/s^2)
Displacement (d, s̄)	meter (m)	Displacement (θ)	radian (rad)
Time (t)	second (s)	Time (t)	second (s)

Since division is not associative, the solidus must not be repeated in the same expression. Ambiguity is avoided by parentheses or by the use of negative powers.

Examples:
m/s^2 or m·s^{-2} (but not m/s/s)
ml/kg·min^{-1}, ml/·kg^{-1}·min, or ml/kg·min (but not ml/kg/min)

When names of units are used, multiplication is indicated simply by a space; the hyphen should not be used.

Examples:
newton meter (not newton-meter or newton·meter)
newton second (not newton-second or newton·second)

When names of units are used, division is indicated by the word "per", and not the solidus

Example:
newton meters per kilogram (not newton meters/kilogram)

Names and Symbols of SI Units

The symbols for SI units remain unaltered in the plural and are written without a final full stop (period) except at the end of a sentence. A space should be left between a numerical value and the first letter of the symbol.

Example:
400 N·m (not 400N·m)

In text, symbols should be used when associated with a number; when no number is involved, however, the unit should be spelled out.

Examples:
The peak torque was 370 N·m (not 370 newton meters)
Peak torque was measured in newton meters (not in N·m)

Names and symbols should not be mixed.

Example:
N·m or newton meter (but not N meter or newton m)

Mass and Weight

The SI units for mass and weight are the kilogram (kg) and the newton (N), respectively. It is almost conventional to use the terms mass and weight interchangeably; in particular, it is common to refer to an individual's body mass in kilograms as a measure of weight. In strict terms, this is not proper use of the term "weight". The weight of an object is equal to its mass multiplied by the acceleration due to gravity. Thus:

$$W = mg$$

where W is weight, m is mass, and g is the acceleration due to gravity (9.80665 m/s^2)

Example:
An individual with a body mass of 70 kg would have a body weight of 686.5 N (70 kg × 9.80665 m/s^2). Popular usage notwithstanding, the distinction between mass and weight should be kept in mind when reporting the results of strength and power measurements.

Conversion to and from SI Units

It would be proper to express the results of tests in SI units; it may be helpful to athletes and coaches, however, also to express the results in other units which are still in common use. Conversions are presented in Table 3.2.

Reproducibility of Measurements

The term "reproducibility", also called "reliability", refers to the amount of variation that occurs in test results between trials in one testing session, or in the results between two or more different days of testing. For example, if you give an athlete two trials at a strength test, what is the variation in the performance on the two trials? Or, if you test the subject on two different days, what is the day-to-day variation?

There are two main sources of variation: (1) biological variation, that is, the relative consistency with which a subject can perform; (2) "experimental error", that is, variations in the way the tests are conducted. An attempt should be made to keep experimental error to a minimum by standardizing the test procedures as described above.

It is a good practice to determine the reproducibility of a measurement before using it on a wide scale. Three methods of determining reproducibility are presented below.

1. Standard Deviation of Repeated Trials

This method may be applied to several trials in one testing session or to the results of several days of testing. It is illustrated in Figure 3.19. The standard deviation (SD) indicates the spread or

Table 3.2   Conversion to and from SI units

Force
1 N = 0.1020 kp (kilopond)†
1 N = 0.2248 lb (pound)*
1 N = 0.1020 kgf (kilogram-force)
1 kp = 9.80665 N
1 lb = 4.448222 N
1 kgf = 9.80665 N

Torque
1 N·m. = 0.737562 ft·lb
1 N·m = 0.101972 kg·m
1 N·m = 0.101972 kp·m
1 ft·lb = 1.355818 N·m
1 kg·m = 9.80665 N·m
1 kp·m = 9.80665 N·m

Linear Displacement
1 m = 3.28084 ft
1 m = 39.37 in
1 ft = 0.3048 m
1 in = 0.0254 m

Linear Velocity
1 m/s = 3.28084 ft/s
1 m/s = 2.236936 mph
1 ft/s = 0.3048 m/s
1 mph = 0.44704 m/s

Power
1 W = 0.00134 hp
1 W = 6.12 kp·m/min
1 W = 0.01433 kcal/min
1 W = 0.06 kJ/min
1 hp = 746 W
1 kp·m/min = 0.163399 W
1 kcal/min = 69.784 W

Work and Energy
1 kJ = 0.238846 kcal
1 J = 0.737562 ft·lb
1 kcal = 4.1868 kJ
1 ft·lb = 1.355818 J

Weight
1 N = 0.101972 kp
1 N = 0.101972 kg
1 N = 0.224809 lb*
1 kp = 9.80665 N
1 kg = 9.80665 N
1 lb = 4.448222 N

Mass
1 kg = 2.204784 lb*
1 lb = 0.45359237 kg

Angular Displacement
1 rad = 57.29578°
1° = 0.017453 rad

Angular Velocity
1 rad/s = 57.29578°/s
1 rad/s = 9.549297 rpm
1°/s = 0.017453 rad/s
1 rpm = 0.10472 rad/s
1°/s = 0.166667 rpm
1 rpm = 6°/s

†The kilopond, a unit of force, is defined as the weight of a 1 kg mass.
*In the British system, mass and force may be expressed in pounds and poundals (absolute system), respectively, or in slugs and pounds (gravitational system), respectively. In the gravitational system, the unit of force, the pound, is defined as the weight of the standard pound (the one pound mass of the absolute system).

dispersion of approximately 70% of the trials; thus, it is a useful indication of the variation in the results. The SD may be expressed in the units of measurement; this expression is meaningful, however, only if the reader is aware of typical test results. For example, a SD of 5 N·m for peak torque measurements would indicate "good" reproducibility if typical average values were 200 N·m, but would indicate "poor" reproducibility if typical test values were 20 N·m. To obviate this problem, the SD is usually expressed as a percentage of the mean test result. The SD expressed this way is called the coefficient of variation (V). The V provides a universal "currency" for expressing reproducibility; that is, the reproducibility of various kinds of measurements can be compared.

A disadvantage of the SD method is that it is an imposition on the subject to make many trials (and in strength testing, there is the problem of fatigue) or to come in for testing on many days. It would also be very time consuming to perform this method on several subjects.

2. Method Error of Repeated Measurements

This method may be applied to two trials in a testing session or to the results of two testing sessions on separate days (Thorstensson, 1976; Friman, 1977). The method is illustrated in Figure 3.20. The method error (ME) may be expressed in the units of measurement or, for the reasons discussed above in relation to the SD method, as a coefficient of variation. The main advantage of the ME over the SD method is that the former is more economical of time for both the subjects and the investigator.

3. Test-Retest Correlation

This method may be applied to two trials in a

REPRODUCIBILITY

MEASURE: ELBOW EXTENSION ON CYBEX AT 30°/s

SUBJECT: RUE SNODGRASS

DAY	PEAK TORQUE, N·m BEST OF 3 TRIALS
1	52
2	48
3	55
4	50
5	47
6	55
7	46
8	53
9	45
10	54
$\overline{X}$ =	50·5
SD =	3·8
V =	7·5%

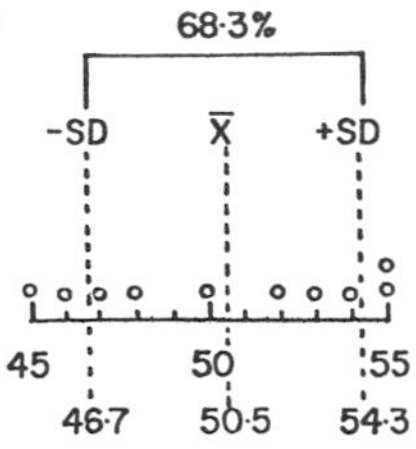

$V = SD/\overline{X} \times 100$

$\overline{X}$ = MEAN
SD = STANDARD DEVIATION
V = COEFFICIENT OF VARIATION

Fig. 3.19. Reproducibility: standard deviation of repeated trials. In this example elbow extension strength was measured on ten different days. The day-to-day variation was expressed as the standard deviation (SD) of the mean of the ten test results. The SD usually is expressed as a coefficient of variation (V). To the right is shown the distribution of the ten test results. The SD indicates the spread of approximately 70% of the test results.

REPRODUCIBILITY

MEASURE: ELBOW EXTENSION AT 30°/s

	SUBJECT	DAY 1 PEAK TORQUE, N·m (BEST OF 3 TRIALS)	DAY 2	DIFF (D)
1	GS	42·0	40·7	1·3
2	RN	50·2	51·5	-1·3
3	TT	40·7	47·5	-6·8
4	MA	48·8	50·2	-1·4
5	CV	47·5	52·9	-5·4
6	SB	63·7	57·0	6·7
7	MC	63·7	61·0	2·7
8	MS	50·2	50·2	0·0
9	BC	42·0	38·0	4·0
10	WC	39·3	47·5	-8·2
	$\overline{X}$ =	48·8	49·7	-0·9 ($\overline{D}$)
	SD =	8·8	6·9	4·8
	SE =	2·8	2·2	1·5

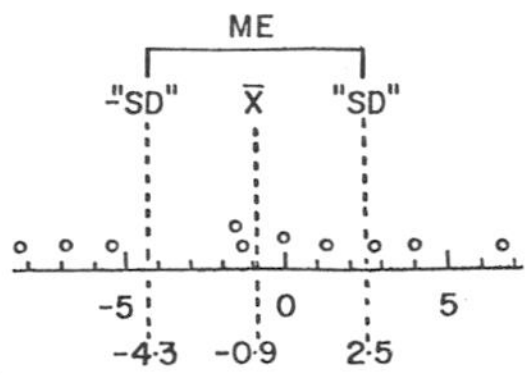

$t = 0·6$ (NS)

$$\text{METHOD ERROR ("SD")} = \sqrt{\frac{\Sigma(D-\overline{D})^2}{2(N-1)}}$$

$$= SD/\sqrt{2}$$

$$= 4·8/1·414$$

$$= 3·4$$

$$V = \frac{ME}{(\overline{X}_1 + \overline{X}_2)/2} \times 100 = \frac{3·4}{49·3} \times 100 = 6·9\%$$

Fig. 3.20. Reproducibility: method error. In this example, ten subjects had their elbow extension strength measured on two different occasions. In each subject, the Day 2 result was subtracted from the Day 1 result. The mean difference was -0.9 N·m. The SD of the mean difference was 4.8 N·m. This value divided by the square root of 2 yields the "method error" (Thorstensson, 1976; Friman, 1977) (ME = 3.4 N·m). The ME usually is expressed as a coefficient of variation (V); that is, as a percentage of the combined means of the two test days: (48.8 + 49.7) /2 = 49.3 N·m; see bottom of figure). This method of determining reproducibility has a built-in check for systematic difference in test results. The standard error of the mean difference (SE = 1.5) divided into the mean difference (-0.9) gives a t ratio (sign ignored) of 0.6 for a "paired" t test. This t ratio indicates that there was no statistically significant difference between the mean values for the two testing sessions.

testing session or to the results of two testing sessions on separate days. In Figure 3.21, the method is illustrated using the same data that were used in Figure 3.20. The closer the correlation coefficient (r) is to 1.0, the better the reproducibility of the measurement.

One disadvantage of this method is that the correlation coefficient is very sensitive to the range of the values used in the computation. Thus, both relatively high and relatively low coefficients may be associated with a similar variation in test results (Figure 3.22). This effect of the range of the data often is unrecognized in the interpretation of correlation coefficients (Clarkson et al., 1980). A second disadvantage of this method is that it does not provide a clear indication of the percent variation (trial-to-trial or day-to-day) in the measurement.

Analysis and Reporting of Results

All of the factors which should be considered in the analysis and reporting of test results have been discussed above. These factors will now be summarized by a series of questions. After each question, the pages on which the factor has been discussed are given.

1. What was the purpose of the test? (p. 13-14)
2. Should the results be expressed absolutely

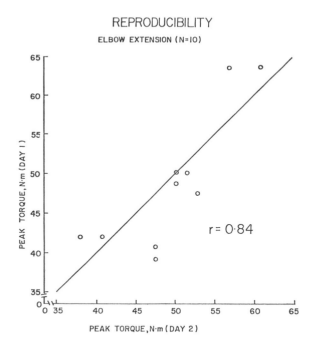

REPRODUCIBILITY

ELBOW EXTENSION (N=10)

$r = 0.84$

Fig. 3.21. Reproducibility: test-retest correlation. The data from the previous figure have been plotted (Day 1 result against Day 2 result). If the reliability were perfect ($r = 1.0$), all data points would lie on the line of identity. In fact, the correlation was $r = 0.84$, and the standard error of the estimate was 5.1 N·m or 10.4% of an average value.

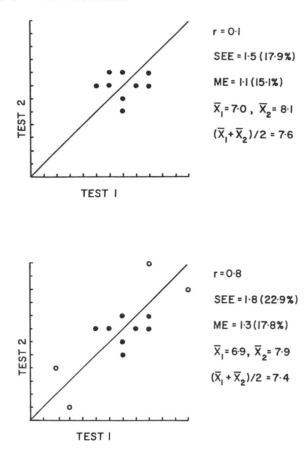

$r = 0.1$

$SEE = 1.5 (17.9\%)$

$ME = 1.1 (15.1\%)$

$\bar{X}_1 = 7.0 , \bar{X}_2 = 8.1$

$(\bar{X}_1 + \bar{X}_2)/2 = 7.6$

$r = 0.8$

$SEE = 1.8 (22.9\%)$

$ME = 1.3 (17.8\%)$

$\bar{X}_1 = 6.9, \bar{X}_2 = 7.9$

$(\bar{X}_1 + \bar{X}_2)/2 = 7.4$

Fig. 3.22. A disadvantage of the test-retest correlation method. Top: In 9 subjects, Test 1 results are plotted against Test 2 results. Because the range of values is small, the correlation coefficient (r) is small (0.10). The method error (ME) calculated from the same data was 15.1%, and the standard error of the estimate (SEE) was 17.9%. Bottom: the results in four more subjects (open circles) are added. The additions increase the range in the results and cause a large increase in the correlation coefficient (0.8); the ME and SEE, however, were not significantly altered (in fact, they are slightly greater). Thus, the correlation coefficient may not provide an accurate indication of test-to-test variation in results.

or per kilogram body mass? (p. 9, 11)

3. In fatigue tests, is the fatigue index or total work done more important? (p. 19, 22, 29)

4. Do the changes observed after training fall within the expected range? (p. 11, 13-14)

5. Is the transfer of training-induced increases in strength and power to performance within the expected range? (p. 14)

6. Have your tests employed a different mode (e.g., isokinetic dynamometer) than the mode (e.g., weight training) with which the athletes trained? (p. 13-14)

7. Do the test-to-test variations you have observed fall within or outside the "reproducibility range" established for your tests? (p. 31-33)

FEE STRUCTURE

Establishing the Fee Structure

Several factors should be considered in the establishment of a fee structure.

Specific Equipment Construction

Specific strength and power testing for a sport will in most cases require a special frame to be constructed to be used with a dynamometer or weights. Materials and technician time should be considered in setting the fee for this construction. It could be a contract separate from regular testing or the cost could be incorporated, over a period of time, into the cost of testing.

Equipment Set-up and Supplies

Technician time is required to set up the equipment prior to a testing session, and also to dismantle it when the session is over. It should be considered that the cost of set-up and dismantling is a relatively smaller proportion of the total cost as the group of athletes tested becomes larger.

The cost of supplies (e.g., recording paper) should be included in the total cost, as well as general overhead costs.

Test Administration

The cost of test administration is directly proportional to the time required to conduct the tests. The number of test movements, the velocities selected (if applicable), and the selection of a fatigue test (if applicable) are the variables which will affect the time required to test an athlete.

Data Analysis

The cost of data analysis also is proportional to the time spent conducting the analysis. Of course, direct computer analysis of the data will be economical in terms of time, but the hourly rate may be higher. Hand calculations from recording paper are very time consuming and in the long run are probably much more expensive than computer analysis.

Time also is required to prepare tables of results and to perform statistical analysis. Again, these tasks are expedited by computer analysis.

Interpretation and Reporting of Test Results

Most of the foregoing can be conducted by trained technicians and assistants. The interpretation and reporting of results usually (and perhaps should always) fall to the sport scientist. This process routinely involves scrutiny of the summarized results, comparison with previous test results, and recommendation of future action on the basis of results. A written report normally is prepared for submission to the coach(es) and athlete(s).

Consultation

The written report may be supplemented with various levels of consultation, the time for which should be considered in establishing the fee.

Sample Fee Structure

By way of clarification, a hypothetical example of a fee structure for the strength and power testing of rowers is given below. It should be recognized that the estimated costs (prepared in 1982) will soon be outdated; nevertheless, the example may be helpful in the establishment of a fee structure. The example is a testing session for a group of ten elite rowers. From a previous contract ($2,000.00), a rowing frame was constructed to permit isokinetic, velocity specific tests. The frame allowed coupling to a Cybex with a gear ratio which tripled the torque capacity (to 1500 N·m) of the instrument. The apparatus included a ratchet mechanism which permitted a rapid, unresisted return stroke suitable for a fatigue test.

(1) Arrangements, co-ordination, and supervision
   The sport scientist is responsible for these:
   5 h @ $50/h $250.00
(2) Equipment set-up and dismantling
   Equipment set-up:
   1 h @ $10/h . . . . $ 10.00
   Equipment dismantling:
   1 h @ $10/h . . . . $ 10.00
   — conducted by technicians or assistants
(3) Administration of tests
   i) Strength and power measurement at specific velocity, simulated rowing movement:
   6 min per athlete for 10 athletes @ $10/h . . . . $ 10.00
   ii) Two-minute fatigue test:
   6 min per athlete for 10 athletes @ $10/h . . . . $ 10.00
   — conducted by technicians or assistants
(4) Data analysis
   i) Data reduction (non-computer) from recordings:
   1 h/athlete for 10 athletes @ $10/h $100.00
   ii) Preparing tables and statistical analysis:
   5 h @ $10/h . . . . $ 50.00
   — conducted by technicians and assistants

(5) Interpretation, reporting, and
    consultation
    i) Preparing written report:
        3 h at $50/h $150.00
    ii) On-site consultation with
        athletes and coaches:
        1 h @ $50/h .... $ 50.00
    — conducted by sport scientist
(6) Estimated general overhead $160.00
              Total $800.00

Cost per athlete: $800/10 = $80.00

REFERENCES

Alderman, R.B. and T.J. Banfield. Reliability estimation in the measurement of strength. *Res. Quart.* 40(3): 448-455, 1969.

Anderson, M.B., R.W. Coté III, E.F. Coyle and F.B. Roby. Leg power, muscle strength and peak EMG activity in physically active college men and women. *Med. Sci. Sports* 11(1): 81, 1979.

Barnes, W.S. The relationship of motor-unit activation to isokinetic muscular contraction at different contractile velocities. *Phys. Ther.* 60(9): 1152-1158, 1980.

Berger, R.A. Determination of a method to predict 1-RM chin and dip from repetitive chins and dips. *Res. Quart.* 38: 330, 1967.

Berger, R.A. *Applied Exercise Physiology.* Lea and Febiger, Philadelphia, 1982.

Brown, C.H. and J.H. Wilmore. The effects of maximal resistance training on the strength and body composition of women athletes. *Med. Sci. Sports* 6(3): 174-177, 1974.

Burke, R.E. and V.R. Edgerton. Motor unit properties and selective involvement in movement. In: *Exercise and Sport Sciences Reviews.* Ed. J.F. Keogh and J.H. Wilmore. New York: Academic Press, 1975, pp. 31-33.

Clarke, H.H. *Muscular Strength and Endurance in Man.* Englewood Cliffs, New Jersey: Prentice-Hall Inc., 1966.

Clarkson, P.M., W. Kroll, and T.C. McBride. Plantar flexion fatigue and muscle fibre type in power and endurance athletes. *Med. Sci. Sports Exercise* 12(4): 262-267, 1980.

Coyle, E.F., D.L. Costill and G.R. Lesmes. Leg extension power and muscle fibre composition. *Med. Sci. Sports* 11(1): 12-15, 1979.

Currier, D.P. Positioning for knee strengthening exercises. *Phys. Ther.* 57(2): 148-152, 1977.

Edington, D.W. and V.R. Edgerton. *The Biology of Physical Activity.* Boston: Houghton Mifflin Co., 1976.

Fisher, M.B. and J.E. Birren. Age and strength. *J. Appl. Psychol.* 31: 490-497, 1947.

Hulten, B., A. Thorstensson, B. Sjodin and J. Karlsson. Relationship between isometric endurance and fibre types in human leg muscles. *Acta Physiol. Scand.* 93: 135-138, 1975.

Ikai, M. and T. Fukunaga. Calculation of muscle strength per unit cross-sectional area of human muscle by means of ultrasonic measurement. *Int. Z. Angew. Physiol.* 26: 26-32, 1963.

Ikai, M. and A.H. Steinhaus. Some factors modifying the expression of human strength. *J. Appl. Physiol.* 16: 157-163, 1961.

Katch, F.I., W.D. McArdle, G.S. Pechar and J.J. Perrine. Measuring leg force-output capacity with an isokinetic dynamometer-bicycle ergometer. *Res. Quart.* 45(1): 86-91, 1974.

Komi, P.V. Relationship between muscle tension, EMG and velocity of contraction under concentric and eccentric work. In: New Developments in *Electromyography and Clinical Neurophysiology, Vol. I.* Basel: Karger, p. 596-606, 1973.

Komi, P.V. and J. Karlsson. Skeletal muscle fibre types, enzyme activities and physical performance in young males and females. *Acta Physiol. Scand.* 103: 210-218, 1978.

Komi, P.V. and J.T. Viitasalo. Changes in motor unit activity and metabolism in human skeletal muscle during and after repeated eccentric and concentric contractions. *Acta Physiol. Scand.* 100: 246-254, 1977.

Kroemer, K.H.E. and J.M. Howard. Towards standardization of muscle strength testing. *Med. Sci. Sports* 2(4): 224-230, 1970.

Lindh, M. Increase of muscle strength from isometric quadriceps exercises at different knee angles. *Scand. J. Rehab. Med.* 11: 33-36, 1979.

MacDougall, J.D., G.C.B. Elder, D.G. Sale, J.R. Moroz and J.R. Sutton. Effects of strength training and immobilization on human muscle fibres. *Eur. J. Appl. Physiol.* 43: 25-34, 1980.

MacDougall, J.D., D.G. Sale, J.R. Moroz, G.C.B. Elder, J.R. Sutton and H. Howald. Mitochondrial volume density in human skeletal muscle following heavy resistance training. *Med. Sci. Sports* 11(2): 164-166, 1979.

Milner-Brown, H.S., R.B. Stein and R.G. Lee. Synchronization of human motor units: possible roles of exercise and supraspinal reflexes. *Electroencephalogr. Clin. Neurophysiol.* 38: 245-254, 1975.

Montoye, H.J. and D.E. Lamphiear. Grip and arm strength in males and females, age 10 to 69. *Res. Quart.* 48: 109-120, 1977.

Moritani, T. and H.A. deVries. Neural factors versus hypertrophy in the time course of muscle strength gain. *Am. J. Phys. Med.* 58: 115-130, 1979.

Murray, D.A., E. Harrison and G.A. Wood. Cybex II reliability and validity: an appraisal. *Med. Sci. Sports Exercise* 14(2): 153, 1982.

Nelson, A.J., M.T. Moffroid, and R. Whipple. The relationship of integrated electromyographic discharge to isokinetic contractions. In Desmedt, J. (ed): *New Developments in Electromyography and Clinical Neurophysiology.* Basel: S. Karger, 1973, pp 584-595.

Olds, K., C.M. Godfrey, and P. Rosenrot. Computer assisted isokinetic dynamometry: a calibration study. Proceedings of the *4th Annual Conference on Rehabilitation Engineering.* Washington, D.C., 1981.

O'Shea, J.P. *Scientific Principles and Methods of Strength Fitness.* Reading, Massachusetts: Addison-Wesley, 1969.

Perrine, J.J. Isokinetic exercise and the mechanical energy potential of muscle. *J. Health. Phys. Educ. Rec.* 39: 40-48, 1968.

Perrine, J.J. and V.R. Edgerton. Muscle force-velocity and power-velocity relationships under isokinetic loading. *Med. Sci. Sports* 10(3): 159-166, 1978.

Pyke, F.S., B.R. Minikin, L.R. Woodman, A.D. Roberts and T.G. Wright. Isokinetic strength and maximal oxygen uptake of trained oarsmen. *Can. J. Appl. Sport Sci.* 4(4): 277-279, 1979.

Rodgers, K.L. and R.A. Berger. Motor unit involvement and tension during maximum, voluntary concentric, eccentric and isometric contractions of the elbow flexors. *Med. Sci. Sports* 6: 253-259, 1974.

Sale, D. and D. MacDougall. Specificity in strength training: a review for the coach and athlete. *Can. J. Appl. Sports Sci.* 6(2): 87-92, 1981.

Sapega, A.A., J.A. Nicholas, D. Sokolow, and A. Saraniti. The nature of torque "overshoot" in Cybex isokinetic dynamometry. *Med. Sci. Sports Exercise* 14(5): 368-375, 1982.

Secher, N.H. Isometric rowing strength of experienced and inexperienced oarsmen. *Med. Sci. Sports* 7(4): 280-283, 1975.

Sharp, R.L., J.P. Troup and D.L. Costill. Relationship between power and sprint freestyle swimming. *Med. Sci. Sports Exercise* 14(1): 53-56, 1982.

Sprague, K. *The Gold's Gym Book of Strength Training for Athletes*. Los Angeles: J.P. Tarcher, Inc, 1979.

Tesch, P. and J. Karlsson. Isometric strength performance and muscle fibre type distribution in man. *Acta Physiol. Scand.* 103: 47-51, 1978.

Thorstensson, A. Muscle strength, fibre types and enzyme activities in man. *Acta Physiol. Scand.* Suppl. 443, 1976.

Thorstensson, A., G. Grimby and J. Karlsson. Force-velocity relations and fiber composition in human knee extensor muscles. *J. Appl. Physiol.* 40: 12-16, 1976.

Thorstensson, A. and J. Karlsson. Fatigability and fibre-composition of human skeletal muscle. *Acta Physiol. Scand.* 98: 318-322, 1976.

Thornton, N. and E.R. Flavell. Dryland performance assessment with isokinetic instrumentation. *Swimming World* 18: 36-39, 1977.

Tornvall, G. Assessment of physical capabilities. *Acta Physiol. Scand.* Suppl. 201, 1963.

Upton, A.R.M. and P.F. Radford. Motoneurone excitability in elite sprinters. In: *Biomechanics V-A*. Ed. P.V. Komi. Baltimore: University Park Press, 1975, 82-87.

Vandervoort, A.A., D.G. Sale and J.R. Moroz. Strength-velocity relation in a bilateral leg press movement. *Med. Sci Sports Exercise* 13(2): 87, 1981.

Wilmore, J. Alterations in strength, body composition and anthropometric measurements consequent to a 10-week weight training program. *Med. Sci. Sports* 6: 133-138, 1974.

Winter, D.A., R.P. Wells and G.W. Orr. Errors in the use of isokinetic dynamometers. *Eur. J. Appl. Physiol.* 46: 397-408, 1981.

CHAPTER FOUR | Testing Aerobic Power

J.S. Thoden • B.A. Wilson • J.D. MacDougall

INTRODUCTION

As summarized in Chapter 2, the energy for muscular contraction during physical exercise is produced from three interdependent sources:

1. The splitting of the high energy phosphates Adenosine Triphosphate (ATP), which is stored at the contractile site and is immediately available for contraction, and Creatine Phosphate (CP), which is immediately available to regenerate the ATP that has been broken down in supporting contraction;

2. Glycolysis, which is the anaerobic breaking down of carbohydrates (glycogen and glucose) to pyruvic or lactic acid; and

3. The aerobic generation of energy, which involves the oxidation of pyruvic acid or fats.

All three processes may occur concurrently, and the proportion of energy derived from each will vary according to the intensity of the exercise. Maximum aerobic power may therefore be considered as being the maximum rate at which energy can be released from the oxidative process exclusively.

The rate at which this process can occur is dependent upon two factors: the chemical ability of tissues to use oxygen in breaking down fuels (peripheral component), and the combined abilities of the pulmonary, cardiac, blood, vascular, and cellular mechanisms to transport oxygen to the aerobic machinery of muscle (central component). Which of these two components is more limiting or more trainable in the athlete is yet unknown. Although it is theoretically possible to isolate either of these components experimentally, the usual measurements of aerobic function avoid these problems by treating transport and utilization as a single unit, and by simply measuring the total amount of oxygen which can be consumed.

Maximum Aerobic Power

Maximum aerobic power can therefore be quantitatively represented as the maximum amount of oxygen which can be consumed per unit of time by a person during a progressive exercise test to exhaustion. It is normally expressed as the volume (V) per minute (V) of oxygen (O_2) which can be consumed by the organism at the maximum (max) workload which can be sustained for a criterion period of time and represented as "VO_2 max".

The value is represented as a volume per minute ($\ell \cdot min^{-1}$) where total power output is important, as in rowing or cycling, and as a volume per kilogram of body weight ($ml \cdot kg^{-1} \cdot min^{-1}$) in activities such as running or nordic skiing where the athlete supports his body weight. Factors affecting maximum aerobic power, such as the oxygen carrying capacity of the blood, the heart, and the pulmonary system are considered elsewhere in this manual.

Nearly all of these processes and capacities can be improved through properly designed training programs. Generally, successful athletes participating in sports which demand sustained effort in excess of two minutes possess much higher aerobic powers than those from shorter or intermittent type sports. The highest values per unit of body weight are demonstrated by nordic skiers and middle distance runners. The highest absolute values generally are demonstrated by athletes such as rowers and cyclists, who also employ a large muscle mass for extended periods, but whose body weight is externally supported.

The extent to which the high aerobic powers of such athletes may be attributed to training rather than to genetic endowment is not known. It has been repeatedly demonstrated, however, that healthy young relatively untrained adults can gain increases of 15% to 20% or more depending on the starting level (Saltin, 1968; Roskam, 1967; Ekblom, 1968; Kasch, 1973; Pollock, 1973; Hollman, 1976). It has also been demonstrated that such increases are due to changes within both the *central* and the *peripheral* components of the aerobic systems (Rowell, 1974).

The Anaerobic Threshold

It is well known that lactic acid will begin to accumulate in the blood of the exercising athlete at work intensities which elicit less than maximal oxygen uptake. Although explanations for this phenomenon vary, in the simplest analysis it is the result of an imbalance between the lactic acid produced by certain muscle fibers contracting anaerobically and the capability of the body to convert or remove it. As the exercise intensity increases, this imbalance is exaggerated, and progressively more and more lactate accumulates in the blood (MacDougall, 1977).

The power output at which blood levels of lactic acid begin to rise significantly above normal resting levels during exercise of increasing intensity has been termed the *anaerobic threshold* (AT). It is generally accepted that an athlete's AT is a very critical factor in determining his potential for sustaining prolonged physical exercise at a high percentage of his $\dot{V}O_2$ max. It is also known that the AT can be elevated through training (Ekblom et al., 1968, Davis et al., 1979) and that successful long-distance athletes have significantly higher thresholds than do normal individuals (Costill, 1970; MacDougall, 1977). It has also been demonstrated recently that, in distance runners, the running velocity at AT is closely related to performance capacity (Farrell et al., 1979; Sjödin and Jacobs, 1981).

Although AT theoretically should be an important parameter to be measured in the long-distance athlete, there are a number of problems associated with interpretation and measurement technique. These will be discussed later in the chapter.

PURPOSES OF TESTING AEROBIC POWER

Periodic and regular testing of aerobic capacity can help determine —
1. the suitability of an athlete for a given type of sport or a specific role in a sport;
2. the emphasis which should be placed on aerobic training;
3. the type of aerobic training which should be employed;
4. the effect of a given program on maximal aerobic power.

In addition, this type of information may assist in determining —
5. the rate at which an athlete is improving, or the rate at which a program is eliciting change;
6. the pattern or pace at which an athlete should compete;
7. whether an athlete is suffering some decline in capacity due to growth, nutritional, or medical factors.

RELEVANCE

Relevance of Maximal Aerobic Power

Evaluation of an athlete's capacity for deriving energy from an aerobic source will be relevant only in those sports and events where performance could be affected by limitations in the process. Thus, measurement of an athlete's aerobic capacity would be of lesser value in predicting his competitive potential if the sport requires a maximal continuous energy expenditure over a time which is less than 40 to 45 s. As the duration of the event becomes greater, aerobic capacity becomes increasingly important as a determining factor for success.

Some activities, such as racquet sports and most team sports, require a series of brief (5 to 20 s) bursts of highly intense energy release separated by periods of lower intensity recovery. Although in such sports most of the energy is directly derived from non-oxidative sources, the recovery portion is an oxidative process. Thus, the rate at which high energy stores can be replaced in the muscles and the by-products of anaerobic metabolism eliminated is to a large extent dependent upon the athlete's maximal aerobic power. Moreover, one could expect the rate of recovery to become a progressively more important factor as the duration of the match or tournament increases. For these reasons, the assessment of maximal aerobic power is also an important test for such athletes.

Examples of sports for which measurement of aerobic power as an indicator of competitive ability would be of greater and lesser value are given in Table 4.1.

Since, quantitatively, $\dot{V}O_2$ max reflects both the

Table 4.1 Relevance of VO₂ max to performance of various sports

HIGHLY RELEVANT	RELEVANT	OF LITTLE RELEVANCE
Track (400 m to marathon)	Alpine Skiing	Jumping and Throwing
Orienteering	Judo	Diving
Swimming (100 m and upwards)	Most Team Sports	Weight Lifting
Cross Country Skiing	Figure Skating	Shooting
	Gymnastics	Archery
Rowing	Canoeing (white water)	Sailing
Canoeing (flat water)	Racquet Sports	Bobsledding
Cycling		Curling
Speed Skating		
Boxing		
Wrestling		

athlete's ability to transport oxygen and his muscles' ability to utilize it, the value will vary according to the mode of exercise and the specific muscles which are involved. Thus, if a measurement of VO₂ max is to be of any practical value to the athlete, the mode of exercise must be controlled and specific to the sport in form, intensity, and duration. Consequently, VO₂ max of runners should be measured on a running treadmill, VO₂ max of rowers should be measured on a rowing ergometer, and so on. Stated in other terms, a measurement of VO₂ max of a swimmer pedalling on a bicycle ergometer is of little practical value in assessing his state of training for swimming.

Relevance of the Anaerobic Threshold

In long-duration endurance events, the ability of an athlete to sustain exercise at a high percentage of VO₂ max may be equal in importance to the actual VO₂ max. Theoretically, measurement of the anaerobic threshold, or that point where blood lactate begins to accumulate, should provide an indication of this ability. When exercise intensity exceeds this level, endurance time is reduced, because of such factors as increased acidity in muscle, and a diminished capacity to mobilize lipids and therefore to spare muscle glycogen (MacDougall, 1977).

It should be noted, however, that depletion of muscle glycogen stores becomes a limiting factor only in the longer distance events and would not likely occur in those events which require less than

30 min to complete. Consequently, measurement of AT would be of most relevance to athletes such as marathon runners and the longer-distance cross-country skiers. In middle distance events such as 800 m - 5000 m in track, many swimming events, rowing, and canoeing, where all athletes compete at intensities which exceed their AT and substrate depletion is not a limiting factor, measurement of AT would be of less relevance. It would be of relatively little importance to team sport athletes, or to athletes such as boxers or wrestlers.

INTERPRETATION OF TEST RESULTS

Advances in knowledge of muscle fiber types has had a great impact on the interpretation of aerobic and anaerobic test results. It is known that skeletal muscle is made up of at least two major types of tissue: fast-contracting fibers which are relatively better at providing energy anaerobically, and slow-contracting fibers which are relatively better able to provide energy aerobically. It is also known that the proportion of each fiber type may vary widely from one muscle to another in a given individual, as well as in the same muscle from one individual to another.

A popular assumption is that the distribution and proportion of fiber type may be important in defining the type of sport and event for which a participant is best suited. While it is generally true that those with a slow-fiber predominance do well in endurance activities, examples of fast-fiber-predominant distance runners have been found (Costill, 1976). This is supported by evidence that fast fibers can experience considerable improvement in aerobic function (Gollnick, 1973). It is therefore conceivable that the inheritance of muscle fiber type may be at least as important in defining the type of training program that is used for a given event as it has been assumed to be in selecting an event. For example, the training of fast fibers for endurance activity should probably be approached quite differently than the training of slow fibers, because fast fibers are not recruited until the work intensity is higher than can be maintained for extended periods (Gollnick, 1974). It also might be speculated that slow-fiber-predominant athletes are trainable for high intensity performances. This is more difficult to support with experimental evidence (Gollnick et al., 1972, 1973, 1974) even though examples of both fast-fiber and slow fiber predominant athletes are found in power events (Costill, 1976).

It follows, therefore, that determining maximal aerobic and anaerobic powers in the untrained individual would be helpful in defining the type of training which would be used for best improving endurance in a given athlete. For example, initially high maximal aerobic power in the relatively untrained individual might indicate a predominance of slow fibers, while high anaerobic power might indicate predominance of fast fibers.

When interpreting test results, one must also examine the aerobic and anaerobic components for a given sport. Estimates of the aerobic and anaerobic sources of energy for maximum-demand competitive events of different durations indicate that events of 5 to 10 s are dependent primarily on phosphagens; events of 40 to 60 s depend on anaerobic lactic energy; events of 2 min require almost equal amounts of both anaerobic and aerobic energy; and events of greater than 2 min depend progressively more on aerobic energy (see Table 4.2).

Such generalizations, however, can be misleading in several instances. For example, this approach is useful only for continuous activity. It has little application in events like hockey and soccer which last 2 to 3 h but which are made up of a series of 5 to 20 s bursts of high rates of energy release separated by periods of lower intensity recovery.

Finally, repeated high-intensity efforts will be possible during training or repeated competitive heats only if a sufficiently high aerobic potential has been developed in order to adequately eliminate the by-products of anaerobic metabolism.

Aerobic function can utilize these by-products as fuel for its own energy replacement process and can therefore either extend anaerobic performance or promote a more rapid recovery.

Consequently, it is misleading to consider that very short events require only anaerobic training, while long events require only aerobic training. A common approach to defining the aerobic and anaerobic needs of a particular sport has been to make measurements of the capacities of international performers. Examples of the results from many such surveys are shown in Table 4.3 and provide a general guideline as to the extent to which aerobic training should be emphasized for a given sport. The need for aerobic training is obvious if low aerobic capacities are measured in those aspiring to endurance events. But there are other applications.

Intuitively, if a sport requires less than one minute for performance, and if international competitors usually are found to have a maximum oxygen consumption of 60-65 $ml \cdot kg^{-1} \cdot min^{-1}$, then it is probably not necessary for an athlete who is near an adequate level to concentrate on training the aerobic system (which can be improved only by about 20% when starting from untrained levels). If, however, an athlete in this type of sport has

Table 4.2   Work time partitioned to percentage aerobic/anaerobic contribution

MAXIMUM EFFORT WORK TIME	ANAEROBIC ALACTIC	ANAEROBIC LACTIC	AEROBIC
5 s	85	10	5
10 s	50	35	15
30 s	15	65	20
1 min	8	62	30
2 min	4	46	50
4 min	2	28	70
10 min	1	9	90
30 min	1	5	95
1 h	1	2	98
2 h	1	1	99

Table 4.3   Range of $\dot{V}O_2$ max reported for international athletes in a variety of sports. Units are $ml \cdot kg^{-1} \cdot min^{-1}$

	RANGE	
SPORT	Males	Females
Nordic Skiing	65-95	56-74
Middle Distance Running	70-86	
Distance Running	65-80	55-72
Rowing	58-74	48-68
Cycling	56-72	
Swimming	54-70	48-68
Soccer	50-70	
Figure Skating		42-54
Wrestling	50-70	
Gymnastics	48-74	38-48
Hockey	45-65	
Field Hockey	39-49	
Basketball	45-65	42-54
Football	40-60	
Baseball	40-60	
Untrained	38-52	30-46

Adapted from the National Coaching Certification Program, Level III.

reasonable performance levels and a very low aerobic capacity (i.e., ½ to ⅔ of usually measured values), some benefit could probably be gained by aerobic training.

Continued testing of advances in maximal aerobic power and recovery ability over a given training period should give insight into the effect of the program design. A lack of improvement may mean either an inability to improve or a faulty approach to training. Perhaps continous training of the aerobic system has reached its limit for improvement, and interval training directed at the peripheral component would be more beneficial.

In some instances, the endurance performer who already possesses a very high aerobic power may receive little benefit from continued emphasis on aerobic training. A training program which trains for lactacid tolerance while maintaining aerobic capacity may be the solution. In such a case, continuous monitoring of aerobic capacity would be necessary to assure that it is being maintained.

A lower than desired level of maximal aerobic power in the athlete who relies exclusively on continuous aerobic training may indicate that the training has not been progressive, or that there is a relatively lower proportion of slow muscle fibers. A possible solution might be to emphasize higher intensity training of the aerobic interval type, in order to recruit fast-twitch muscle fiber tissue and

Table 4.4 Some ways to apply test results to training program design

MEASURED $\dot{V}O_2$ MAX	CONDITIONS	SOME POSSIBLE INTERPRETATIONS FOR AEROBIC TRAINING
High	endurance athlete, mixed training	— perhaps limit in central or peripheral component — perhaps training needs progression in intensity — perhaps has reached overall limit and requires move to anaerobic training
High	relatively untrained	— perhaps high slow-fiber proportion, low lean and total body weight, high central component capacity — try continuous training closely followed by aerobic interval
High	relatively well trained (continuous type), poor ability to perform at high % $\dot{V}O_2$ max	— perhaps poor fast-fiber aerobic capacity — try mixed or aerobic interval emphasis — may have reached limit, try anaerobic training with aerobic maintenance and monitoring
Moderate	relatively well trained, continuous type	— perhaps needs progression in intensity — perhaps moderate slow-fiber population — move to aerobic interval training
Moderate	relatively well trained (mixed, or aerobic interval)	— perhaps has reached limit in central component — try emphasizing continuous then aerobic interval
Moderate	relatively untrained	— difficult to assess — try continuous and progress to mixed or aerobic interval
Low	partially trained, continuous type	— perhaps low central or peripheral component — perhaps low slow-fiber proportion — try progression of continuous, or move to aerobic interval
Low	relatively untrained	— difficult to assess — perhaps low slow-fiber proportion — initially continuous, with progression to mixed and aerobic interval
Low	relatively easily gained improvement (mixed aerobic interval)	— perhaps low fast-fiber population — emphasize continuous

Note: The validity of this table —
1) assumes a continuing test-retest program to continually monitor the effectiveness of the approach chosen;
2) depends on the testing of all energy systems;
3) assumes absence of disease and other health or psychological problems.

to initiate its aerobic adaptation.

Further examples of the ways in which a variety of information and test results can be combined to assist in the selection of an approach to training are summarized in Table 4.4.

In summary, there are many ways of employing tests to assist effectively in using individual talents and training time. It also must be stressed that energy generation, storage, and release are interdependent, and that aerobic and anaerobic energy production are simultaneous and continuously occurring processes that fluctuate with demand for energy. A testing program, therefore, for any type and duration of sport is incomplete unless both aerobic and anaerobic processes are evaluated.

TESTING PROCEDURES

A progressive increase in the rate of energy expenditure will result in progressive increases of both aerobic and anaerobic function until finally the aerobic maximum is reached. This maximum is identifiable as the point at which there is no further increase in aerobic energy production or the uptake of oxygen despite further increases in exercise intensity. Any test, therefore, which requires progressively more energy expenditure per unit of time will eventually achieve the aerobic energy maximum, providing it can be continued for a long enough time. Criteria for achieving this will be discussed later.

An industrial approach to measuring energy expenditure might use a dynamometer or a thermally sensitive apparatus. This is either not possible or inconvenient with living organisms because of fluctuating efficiencies in performing physical exercise, and because a certain proportion of the energy is anaerobic and this proportion changes as exercise becomes more intense. An alternative is to measure the amount of oxygen which is used by the system and assume it to be an equivalent for the energy produced aerobically. This is not quite correct because it takes different amounts of oxygen to release an equivalent amount of energy from fat than from sugar. This discrepancy, however, can be overlooked during maximal or near maximal exercise, since the fuel which is utilized is almost exclusively sugar. Thus, the amount of oxygen which is utilized during a maximal test can be considered as an index of the energy produced by the muscle.

Consequently, the athletic world has become accustomed to the use of the term "oxygen consumption" in either absolute units (liters per minute) or relative units (milliliters per kilogram of body weight per minute) to describe aerobic energy production. The point at which the aerobic production ceases to rise following further increases in intensity has become known as the Maximum Aerobic Capacity or *Maximum Oxygen Consumption* ($\dot{V}O_2$ max). Slightly different or more precise terminology may be used in different laboratories, depending on the application.

Aerobic Testing Protocols

The following points must be considered in the design of an aerobic test:

1. The progression of power output must begin at a low enough level to serve as a warm-up. Without this, the aerobic function may accelerate so slowly that lactate accumulates to fatiguing levels before $\dot{V}O_2$ max is attained.

2. The progressive power output increments must be small enough to avoid undue increases in lactate, and large enough so that total test time is not prolonged to the point where depletion of glycogen or elevation of body temperature may prove limiting. Ideally, the final increment will result in an exercise intensity which must be terminated about 60 to 90 s after $\dot{V}O_2$ max has been attained.

3. It is preferable that the type of work, with respect to rate, resistance, muscle mass used, and range of motion, be identical to the participant's competitive activity. Any departure from this approach results in measurements of aerobic power in tissues that are not used, or are used differently than in competition, and gives, at best, a related rather than a specific value. The impact of this criterion is that a "universal" test is not possible; only a generally applicable protocol can be defined. More specifically, runners should be measured while running, rowers while rowing, swimmers while swimming, and so on. Even nonspecific tests, however, have a value in assessing the oxygen transport characteristics. For instance, rowers might be trained in the off-season by running, and an aerobic power test while running would have the value of assessing the central component of the oxygen transport system and the effects of the intervening program.

4. The wide range of maximal aerobic powers found among athletes requires that the selection of increments in power output be variable. Too large a demand on the lower capacity individuals

and the criterion point of maximum aerobic function may be missed; too low an increment and VO_2 max may not be attained before other factors force cessation of the test. For example, a treadmill test where belt speed is too low and which increases the angle of the machine to achieve work increments may result in such a severe angle for the superior athlete that the running style is too different to give valid measures. Conversely, a treadmill test which uses only increased speed as the work increment may exceed the power performer's running capability.

5. Tests for the less well prepared athlete generally demand lower work increments. This very often can be done by a continuous protocol without rest periods between loads. Maximum tests for better athletes usually require such intense exercise that intervals of rest may be required between each load. Such intermittent testing, however, should be completed with a maximum of three or four loads, to avoid premature fatigue or inordinate prolongation of the test.

Predictive Testing

Why use a predictive test? Some or all of the following points may explain why many situations are ideal for predictive assessment of VO_2 max: (1) test duration is usually shorter than that of direct measurement tests; (2) tests can be submaximal (this increases the safety margin, especially for high-risk subjects); (3) tests are relatively inexpensive; (4) minimal equipment is required; (5) lower expertise in testing may be employed; (6) results are immediate; (7) some tests allow for group testing.

Predictions from submaximal exercise data generally are based on the assumptions that a relationship exists between VO_2 and other more easily measured variables during submaximal work, and that extrapolations to maximal work levels can be made to predict the VO_2 max. There is an abundance of these tests in the literature, and only a few basic examples will be given here. For more complete discussions of this type of test, see Åstrand, 1974; Balke, 1960; deVries, 1968; Fox, 1973; Harrison, 1980; Jetté, 1979; or Lange-Anderson, 1971.

One of the most popular techniques involves the measurement of submaximal heart rate (HR) as a predictor. The Åstrand-Rhyming Nomogram (Åstrand, 1974) provides an example of this type of test and is based on the assumptions of a linear

relationship between HR and work load in a progressive test and of a standard relationship between HR and age. Heart rates at two or more known submaximal workloads are entered into tables or a nomogram to predict the VO_2 at an estimated maximum HR, on the assumption that the two variables occur simultaneously under normal circumstances. Error arises in such methods due to inaccuracies in the methods for estimating maximum heart rates and differences in the effect of stress on heart rate within and between athletic and untrained groups. Thus, while such methods are helpful for mass screening programs and sometimes for comparing individuals against themselves over time, they are generally considered a poor basis for the comparison of athletic populations.

Predictions from maximal power output require exercise to exhaustion and assume an efficiency value for the exercise task. They require a minimum of equipment and may allow for group testing. One example of this type of test is the Balke (1960) cycle ergometer test. Exercise begins at 300 kgm·min^{-1} and 50 rpm and continues with 150 kgm·min^{-1} increments every 2 min until exhaustion. The VO_2 max can be calculated for the last power output completed by multiplying the final kgm by 2 ml O_2 and adding 300 ml for resting VO_2. These tests have proven to be reasonably accurate, but they do require maximal output by the subjects, and they do have a tendency to overestimate VO_2 max for highly motivated subjects who may complete a higher power output primarily on anaerobic input.

In summary, although inexpensive and easy to administer, predictive tests are subject to error. For group data, they are excellent, with the error between predicted and measured VO_2 being less than 10%. The range of data can spread, however, to 25% difference for some subjects (Bonen, 1979; Davies, 1968). The type of subject for whom these tests are poor predictors tends to be in the very low or very high VO_2 max categories. It is therefore recommended that any use of predictive tests with elite performers be very carefully administered and interpreted, using only normative data which have been developed from elite athletes of that sport while performing the same test.

Direct Measurement of VO_2 max

Direct measurement protocols generally fall into one of three categories:

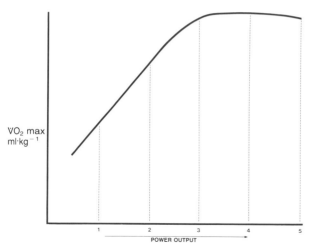

Fig. 4.1   Oxygen uptake ($\dot{V}O_2$) during progressive exercise to exhaustion. In this instance, the $\dot{V}O_2$ at phase 4 indicates $\dot{V}O_2$ max.

1. Continuous progressive loading;
2. Discontinuous progressive loading;
3. Constant loading.

It has been shown that $\dot{V}O_2$ max values determined by each of these protocols will produce the same value in a given individual (McArdle et al., 1973). Attainment of $\dot{V}O_2$ max is assured when a plateau (as indicated by a change <100 ml·min^{-1}) or a slight drop in the $\dot{V}O_2$ occurs as work is increased beyond the work intensity that first results in a maximum value (Figure 4.1). Other information which has been used as criteria to establish that valid $\dot{V}O_2$ max values have been attained includes exhaustion, reaching of the age-predicted maximum HR, an R value in excess of 1.00, and plasma lactate above 10 mM/ℓ.

Constant load tests involve the selection of a workload which will exhaust the subject in greater than 3 but less than 6 min. They therefore rely on maximal criteria factors other than the $\dot{V}O_2$ plateau data to confirm that $\dot{V}O_2$ max has been reached. A great deal of experience and/or a progressive power pretest are required to determine the test load. Although this is a short test, and accurate in the hands of experienced technicians, it is not recommended for general use.

Discontinuous and continuous progressive load tests differ primarily in the method of increasing power output. In the discontinuous protocol, a rest period of set duration is given between loads. Each successive load is much harder, and as many loads as necessary are used until the last load achieves exhaustion between 3 and 6 min. This prolongs the total test time, but does allow for communication with the subject before the next workload, and often allows time for $\dot{V}O_2$ and other calculations even without on-line analytical systems. This mode of testing is useful with subjects who are naïve to treadmill running and where time allows. Continuous progression testing uses a smaller work increment and depends on previous loads to shorten the time that must be spent at the last load (about 1 min) in order to achieve maximum values. Both of these protocols require that the initial load be selected to give a minimum of four measurements during the test in order to allow the use of the "plateau" criterion for identifying $\dot{V}O_2$ max, and both may be used with several modes of exercise, such as those applied to bicycle, running, and arm cranking ergometers.

Treadmill Running

Tests of $\dot{V}O_2$ max on the treadmill traditionally use one of three methods for increasing the exercise intensity:

1. Increasing velocity with elevation kept constant;
2. Increasing elevation with velocity kept constant; and
3. Increasing both elevation and velocity.

One problem which is often encountered when the treadmill is kept level and the velocity is increased is that the test speed might exceed the running skill of the athlete before true maximum criteria can be achieved. Conversely, a test which results in excessive elevation of the treadmill may alter the running mechanics to the extent that its validity is questionable. Although a combination of the two methods is probably the most effective, it results in a more complicated protocol.

An alternative is to select a running speed which will achieve $\dot{V}O_2$ max without increasing the grade excessively. Such a protocol is recommended later in this chapter. It has been found by the authors to be acceptable for athletes from a wide range of sports and to be reliable ($r = 0.95$) when tested in three different laboratories.

Cycle Ergometry

$\dot{V}O_2$ max values elicited on a cycle ergometer are often lower than those found when the same subject is tested on a treadmill (McArdle et al., 1973). Moreover, it is more difficult to demonstrate a plateau in VO_2 in subjects who do not train by cycling. When testing cyclists, however, the ergometer obviously is the most appropriate device.

Arm ergometry. Arm cranking of a cycle ergometer presents one problem not usually encountered with running and cycling: local muscle fatigue. This can cause termination of exercise before any plateau of VO_2 is reached. In order to compensate for this problem, two approaches may be taken. One is to use a discontinuous test, allowing adequate rest periods (5-10 min) for muscle recovery. A second is to reduce the duration of the work periods and decrease the workload increments from the normal 25 W load used for leg work to 12.5 W. Whereas such a test may be appropriate for testing paraplegic athletes, its validity for simulating such sports as swimming or paddling is questionable.

In instances where specific laboratories have the appropriate equipment (i.e., swimming tank, flume, or ergometric apparatus; rowing or paddling ergometer; treadmill modified for arm and leg work as in cross-country skiing, etc.), it is recommended that the basic protocol and criteria described here be incorporated, using the methods of progressive loading which are appropriate to the apparatus.

Summary

When testing VO_2 max of highly trained performers, it is suggested that the following points be considered:

1. Predictive tests may produce large errors in some individuals and populations;

2. The movement pattern of the tests should be matched as precisely as possible to the subject's mode of training and performing;

3. Achieving a plateau should be the ultimate criterion for determining VO_2 max, and therefore some form of progressive workload test should be used.

Measurement of the Anaerobic Threshold

Many European scientists arbitrarily define AT, or the onset of blood lactate, as that point where plasma lactate concentration exceeds $4.0 \ mM \cdot \ell^{-1}$ (see Kindermann et al., 1979 and Skinner and McLellan, 1980). While this provides a definitive and objective criterion for assessing AT, it necessitates invasive serial sampling of blood during a progressive exercise test.

An alternative non-invasive method estimates the AT from alterations in certain respiratory gas exchange parameters. It has been demonstrated (Wasserman et al., 1973 and Davis et al., 1976) that the point of non-linear increases in ventilation (V_E) and carbon dioxide production (VCO_2), in combination with a decline in expired CO_2 tension (F_ECO_2) and an elevation of expired O_2 tension (F_EO_2), shows a good correlation with the point of increase in venous blood lactate.

A number of practical problems arise in attempting to estimate AT from gas exchange measures.

1. The point of non-linearity in a given variable

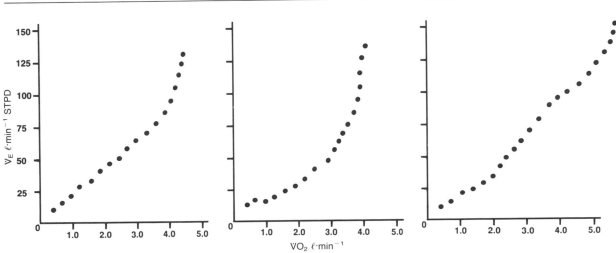

Fig. 4.2 V_E-VO_2 relationship for 3 different subjects during progressive exercise on a bicycle ergometer. Subjects pedalled for 3 min at each workload and V_E was recorded every 30 s. (Human Performance Laboratory, McMaster University)

must be subjectively determined, whether it is graphed against time or workload (e.g., V_E against kpm on a cycle ergometer), or against a second variable (e.g., V_E against VO_2). Although in the majority of subjects who are tested, the point of non-linearity is quite obvious, in many it is not (see Figure 4.2). The authors of this chapter have found the reproducibility of the method on a test-retest basis, or among different investigators, to be rather poor. Davis et al. (1976) acknowledged routine differences among investigators of the estimate of AT which would result in errors in excess of 15%. It therefore becomes questionable whether this method is accurate enough to reflect the slight changes which might occur in the elite athlete over a given training period, or if it provides a reasonable basis for comparing the potential of different athletes.

2. Since the exercise mode must be sport-specific in order for the results to have any practical value for the athlete, a problem is encountered when testing runners. It is of major importance that the linear portion of the response be well established so that a "breakaway" point can be seen. This necessitates measurement of respiratory parameters beginning with very low power outputs (e.g., from 20% VO_2 max onwards). On a treadmill, such speeds are too slow for running, and the subject is forced to walk. Conversely, if the test commences at a proper running speed (e.g., 8 mph) a subject who has a VO_2 max of 65 ml·kg^{-1} already will be exceeding 60% of his VO_2 max.

3. In an attempt to accommodate for the time of diffusion of lactate from the muscle to the plasma, and for the subsequent respiratory response time, some investigators advocate a test which causes the subject to remain at each work level for 3 min (Katch et al., 1978 and McLellan et al., 1981). This results in long total test times and makes it difficult to measure VO_2 max and AT with the same test.

4. Interpretation of AT from respiratory data may be complicated by individual differences in ventilatory sensitivity to CO_2 or H^+ which may affect the relationship between V_E and increases in plasma lactate.

5. There is some question as to which break-point in V_E should be used for estimating AT (Skinner and McLellan, 1980). As well, there is a suggestion that non-linear changes in ventilatory parameters may be just coincidental with the onset of lactic acid accumulation and not a cause-effect relationship (Hagberg et al., 1981 and Davis

and Gass, 1981).

For the above reasons, the authors of this chapter feel that, for the purposes of testing elite athletes, estimates of AT by non-invasive methods should be discouraged.

RECOMMENDED TESTING PROCEDURES

Recommended Treadmill VO_2 max Protocol

A progressive continuous test is recommended at the following constant speeds:
— 7.0 mph for females
— 7.5 mph for female runners
— 8.0 mph for males
— 8.5 mph for male runners

To confirm the achievement of a plateau for VO_2, it is also recommended that the progressive test be followed by a supramaximal constant load test.

Progressive Phase

It is recommended that the test be preceded by a 5 to 10 min accommodation period at a speed determined to be comfortable by the athlete (usually 5.0-7.0 mph).

The time sequence and loading for the test is as follows:

TIME	% GRADE
0 - 2 min	0
2 - 4 min	2
4 - 6 min	4
6 - 8 min	6
8 - 10 min	8
10 - 12 min	10
12 - 14 min	12
etc.	etc.

Exhaustive Phase

Following a 15 min recovery, the subject runs to exhaustion at the last progressive test grade at which a full two minutes of exercise was completed. In subsequent test sessions, subjects who have performed for longer than 6 min during the exhaustive run phase of previous VO_2 max tests should be exercised at a grade which is 2% greater than that completed during the progressive phase of the current test.

This test protocol is also recommended for cross-country skiing and other arm-leg combination ergometers.

Detailed Steps for Administration of the Test

The following protocol is recommended as standard for a treadmill test of VO_2 max:

1. The purpose and procedures of the test are explained to the subject.

2. The subject is prepared with electrodes (V_5) and asked to sign the consent form (Appendix 4.1).

3. Introduction to treadmill running begins at 4.0 mph and gradually is increased to the subject's preferred warm-up speed (usually 5.0-7.0 mph). This is continued for a minimum of 5.0 min, or until the subject is satisfied.

4. Recovery to a heart rate of less than 120 bpm (or longer, if the subject wishes) is allowed.

5. Subjects attaining a heart rate greater than 160 bpm during the warm-up are run at 7.5 mph; of 140 to 160 bpm, at 8.0 mph; of less than 140 bpm, at 8.5 mph. This is variable according to running skill; less skilled runners are run at the next lower speed. A similar approach is used for the bicycle loads.

6. The subject is attached to the breathing apparatus (usually suspended or held by a technician) and begins to run at 0% grade.

7. Measurement of gas variables is made in the last 45 s of each load. Gas volume is determined for a minimum of 30 s.

8. The treadmill angle is increased by 2% of its length each two minutes.

9. If the gas collection is non-continuous, the subject is instructed to advise if the next load will be completed. If he cannot do so, the subject is asked to estimate and advise by hand signals when exercise can be maintained for 30 to 60 s longer. When this signal is made, the final measurement is taken. The test is terminated when the subject grasps the treadmill handrail.

10. The subject is encouraged to "cool down" by resuming moderate exercise at 0% grade and a speed of 4.0 to 5.0 mph for several minutes.

11. The subject is then allowed to recover to a HR of less than 120 bpm (or longer if requested).

12. The same protocol of collection is followed for a run of maximum time at the grade and speed of the last load completed.

13. The calculations are plotted to ascertain that a VO_2 max plateau was reached, and the VO_2 max is taken as the highest value attained in either the progressive or the exhaustive test.

Recommended Cycle Ergometer VO_2 max Protocol

The recommended pedalling rate is 60 rpm for general use and 90 rpm for cyclists.

Exhaustive Phase

After completing the progressive phase, subjects rest 15 min and then complete a ride to exhaustion at a load equal to the last load completed in the progressive phase. In subsequent test sessions, subjects who have completed more than 6 min during the exhaustive phase of previous tests should work at 300 kpm (50 W) above the last load completed in the current progressive phase.

PROGRESSIVE PHASE	EXPECTED VO_2 MAX 3.5 - 4.0 $\ell \cdot MIN^{-1}$	EXPECTED VO_2 MAX 4.0 - 6.0 $\ell \cdot MIN^{-1}$
Time	Power Output	Power Output
0 - 2 min	300 kpm (50 W)	600 kpm (100 W)
2 - 4 min	600 kpm (100 W)	900 kpm (150 W)
4 - 6 min	900 kpm (150 W)	1200 kpm (200 W)
6 - 8 min	1100 kpm (180 W)	1500 kpm (250 W)
8 - 10 min	1300 kpm (215 W)	1800 kpm (300 W)
10 - 12 min	1500 kpm (250 W)	2100 kpm (350 W)
12 - 14 min	1700 kpm (280 W)	2400 kpm (400 W)
etc.	etc.	etc.

Parameters to be Measured

The suggested analysis techniques are covered in the section *Test Equipment*. Measurements are taken continuously or during the last 45 s of each load and for each 45 s interval beyond 1.5 min on the supramaximal load and include V_E or V_I, F_EO_2, F_ECO_2, and HR, from which VO_2, VCO_2, and R may be calculated.

Reliability

Fifteen subjects were tested using the recommended treadmill test (i.e., five subjects at three different laboratories). In all three locations, a basic open circuit system was used. Systems varied, however, in that either a mixing box, bag collection, or Tissot spirometer technique was employed. A test-retest was performed on each of the subjects. The VO_2 max of the subjects tested ranged from 46 ml$\cdot$kg$^{-1}\cdot$min^{-1} to

76 ml·kg^{-1}·min^{-1}. There were no significant differences from test to retest and the Pearson r correlation was 0.95. The greatest lab retest difference for a single subject was 3 ml·kg^{-1}·min^{-1}.

Recommended Protocol for Calculation of Anaerobic Threshold

It is suggested that AT measurement is relevant only for those athletes involved in long-duration events. Although there may be some merit in the assessment of AT for the purpose of training prescription in other athletes, the test should be sport specific, since the level of AT varies according to the mode of exercise (Davis et al., 1976). Thus, measurement of AT in a swimmer while on a treadmill or bicycle ergometer would be of little value in attempting to derive a HR-AT relationship for prescribing training intensity. On the other hand, invasive sampling during a progressive swimming test poses serious logistical problems which would make the test difficult to administer on a routine basis for elite swimmers.

It is recommended —

1. that measurement of AT should be limited to long distance athletes;

2. that AT should be considered as that point, during a progressive exercise test, where plasma lactate reaches a concentration of 4 mM·ℓ^{-1};

3. that venous or arterialized blood be sampled (by fingertip puncture or by means of an indwelling catheter) at rest and during *continuous* exercise at each workload following that at which the subject achieves a pulse rate of 120 bpm;

4. that the mode of exercise be sport-specific and that the protocol be similar to that suggested for VO$_2$ max, but that the subject spend 3 min at each workload and that blood be sampled during the last 30 s of each workload;

5. that the level of the AT be expressed in terms of oxygen uptake (i.e., VO$_2$ at AT or % VO$_2$ max) and pulse rate (i.e., HR at AT);

6. that estimation of AT from respiratory gas exchange parameters is not sufficiently reliable to reflect the minor changes which might occur over a given training period; and that, until further investigation, this method should not be used for the purpose of testing elite athletes.

Test Equipment

Equipment for VO$_2$ max and AT evaluation falls into three categories:

1. Loading (treadmill, bicycle, etc.);
2. Gas collection;
3. Gas analysis.

A large number of manufacturers market equipment in each category, some of which is designed for specialized research or clinical applications, and some of which is unsuitable for athlete testing due to the extreme range of power outputs and ventilatory volumes which may be found in competitive sport. The following is a listing of minimum criteria for testing equipment for aerobic testing of elite athletes.

Loading Equipment

Aside from the cosmetic features, quietness, and durability, the requirements for loading apparatus are —

a) that the loading mechanism be adjustable during operation;

b) that the control mechanism provide a precision of repeated adjustments of less than ± 1% of the testing load, both during the test and between tests;

c) that the physical structure be adjustable to accommodate the smallest and largest athlete comfortably;

d) that the protective characteristics and surrounding arrangement of equipment provide a feeling of security for the subject and operator;

e) that the mechanism for carrying out and verifying the calibration be used easily.

Thus, a treadmill should be set in the floor or surrounded by a platform that provides a wide area of good footing and encloses all moving parts but the belt. It should have a strong support railing at the front and sides which does not restrict movement. It should have a wide scale indication of speed and angle and a separate revolution counter. The walking surface should be not less than 1.8 m × 0.6 m. The braking system for stopping the belt should be variable to allow both immediate and coasting stops. Elevation should be hydraulically or mechanically variable over a range of 0 to 20%. The treadmill should have a mechanical device for verifying the angle of incline. The speed should be infinitely variable from 2.0 mph to 12 mph, and belt revolutions should be counted to verify each speed selected.

A bicycle should be of the constant load variety, with precise metering of revolutions per minute and a revolution counter for calibration. Ideally, the resistance should be electrically controlled between 0 and 3000 kgm (500 W) per minute. Mechanically controlled resistances are used widely but are difficult to read accurately, to adjust precisely during exercise, and to maintain stable with a varying pedalling rate. Handle bars should be vertically and horizontally adjustable, and the saddle should be adjustable for height and angle. Ideally, saddles of the racing, touring, and sprung variety should be available to accommodate preferences. The crank length should be between 16.5 - 17.5 cm and be fitted with toe clips.

Gas Collection Equipment

The primary concerns in constructing a gas collection circuit are that it —

a) be *absolutely* air tight under a pressure loading greater than 1 lb per square inch;

b) provide a resistance to airflow of less than 5 cm H_2O during the transition from 0 flow rate to peak flow rates of 450 $\ell \cdot min^{-1}$ (i.e., not exceed ± 5 cm H_2O pressure in the inspired or expired line in an exercise test during which ventilations exceed 225 $\ell \cdot min^{-1}$);

c) be fitted with valves that allow an interchange between atmospheric and circuit breathing without exceeding the above pressure limits;

d) be fitted with valves that allow interchange in less than 1/10 s;

e) be fitted with a connection to the subject (mouthpiece or face mask) that is comfortable and does not restrict movement or add weight to the subject;

f) be fitted with a direct volume collection system that is of low inertia and is not sensitive to variation as a function of breathing frequency or air flow rate;

g) provide a reading of gas temperature during volume determination;

h) provide a method for mixing a minimum of two breaths (8 ℓ) of gas before gas samples are taken for analysis;

i) provide for absolutely anaerobic collection of gas samples for analysis;

j) be easily dissembled for cleaning and sterilization;

k) allow for collection of a minimum of 30 s of ventilation (at least 110 ℓ) during every minute of testing;

l) provide a gas volume measurement of less than ± 0.05 ℓ error at any volume.

Figure 4.3 is a schema of one such apparatus which is designed for use on the expired side. Inspired-side circuits utilizing a low resistance pneumotachometer are feasible but are generally more expensive to construct and must be pre-calibrated against a range of flow rates. Similarly, inspired volume may be measured with volumetric apparatus, but this offers little advantage since expired gases must still be collected for O_2 and CO_2 analysis.

Mechanical gasometers involve varying degrees of inertial problems which can result in up to 5% error at 100 $\ell \cdot min^{-1}$ of exercise ventilation. Pneumotachographs often are accompanied by resistance or temperature problems which make them subject to mechanical or mathematical corrections if applied to a wide range of exercise ventilations. Collection of gas in large bags increases the opportunity for volume error in subsequent procedures and for contamination of gas samples either by diffusion or addition of dead space gas from connectors. In addition, bag collection provides for no mechanism of rapid or electrical recording of volumes. Thus, while any of these mechanisms can be made to work reasonably well, the potential for error in determining the large volumes associated with maximum exercise by the superior performer makes them somewhat

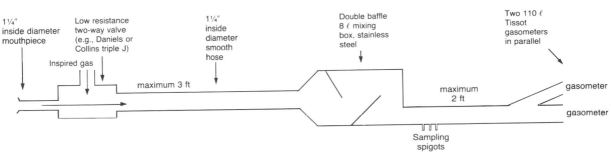

Fig. 4.3 A sample schema for a gas collection system

less reliable. The recommended apparatus, therefore, is a 110 ℓ Tissot flow-through gasometer fitted with a minimum of 1¼″ inside diameter airways.

Gas Analysis Equipment

It is with this equipment that the greatest potential for undetected error rests. Minor errors in adjusting load or in calculating gas volume remain relatively minor, while errors in determining oxygen and carbon dioxide are multiplied in the calculations of VO_2. The following criteria, therefore, are of special importance. The methods for determining oxygen and carbon dioxide concentrations must —

a) give repeated readings within ± 0.02% oxygen content and 0.04% carbon dioxide content (i.e., have a scale that can be read to, and will vary less than, 0.02% and 0.04% respectively, during the time of the test);

b) where applicable, allow transfer of gas sample volume with contamination of less than 0.1% volume (i.e., less than 0.1 ml contamination per liter);

c) if electronic in nature, allow for repeated calibrations at 15 min intervals throughout the test duration.

In addition, electronic apparatus should be supplied by a constant voltage transformer system. Calibration should be done with gas of at least three concentrations: one that approximates the values to be read during the test (15 to 20% O_2 and 3 to 5% CO_2) and one 2 to 3% both above and below this concentration. The calibration gas should be verified with volumetric (Scholander) apparatus at least once each month, and tanks of calibration gas should be exchanged annually.

It is easiest and most reliable to install electronic apparatus which meets these specifications directly in the collection line in order to avoid contamination of the samples. Installation is downstream from the mixing box and through gas drying compounds. In so doing, the flow rate of sample gas and response characteristics of the analyzer should be such that any change in expired gas is detected within 5 s. This response time is not applicable for breath-by-breath analysis but is adequate for measurement of VO_2 max. The precision of this approach depends on averaging the reading throughout the sampling period (through the use of recorders or signal averagers), and in weekly comparisons of these readings with

samples drawn from the gas volume apparatus where the percentage of O_2 and CO_2 for the entire period of collection can be determined. Variation should be within the above specifications.

Calculations

VO_2 is calculated according to the basic formula:

$$VO_2 = (V_I \times F_IO_2) - (V_E \times F_EO_2)$$

The methods of determining $V_{I/E}$ (inspired and expired gas volume per min) and $F_{I/E}O_2$ (fraction of inspired and expired gas which is oxygen) and of expressing them in STPD (Standard Temperature and Pressure, Dry Gas), as well as of calculating the other variables (frequency, respiratory exchange, etc.) are presented in Appendices 4.2, 4.3, 4.4. There are several methods of calculation, which differ slightly; but all are usable if they transform volumes to STPD units, account for differences in inspired and expired volumes, use corrected barometric pressures, and make no assumptions related to the metabolic substrate (fat, protein, or carbohydrate).

Report Form

This will vary according to the test battery which is used, and the degree of interpretation made probably is best left to the laboratory involved. Examples of output forms which present all values in a composite test battery and rank athletes in a group of those tested are shown in Appendices 4.5 and 4.6. These have proven valuable as a basis for interpreting and providing data to coaches.

FEE STRUCTURE

This is a highly variable item, and only very general guidelines can be constructed.

a) A single test is likely to involve 1½ h, including calculations and plotting.

b) A single test is likely to involve two technicians.

c) Interpretation is likely to involve a minimum of ½ h with the coach.

d) Laboratory space and equipment cannot be used for the period of the test and require maintenance and renewal proportional to their use.

The best estimates from three laboratories for the above operational and capital expenses in an existing laboratory for a single test are:

(1) Personnel
        execution . . . . $ 50.00
        interpretation . . . . $ 20.00
(2) Supplies. $ 10.00
(3) Maintenance, etc. . . . . $ 20.00

                    Per subject $100.00

Most laboratories should be able to conduct group tests (five or more subjects) for one-half to two-thirds of this cost.

REFERENCES

Åstrand, P., and I. Rhyming. A nomogram for calculation of aerobic capacity from pulse rate during submaximal work. *J. Appl. Physiol.* 7:218-221, 1954.

Åstrand, P.O., K. Rodahl. *Textbook of Work Physiology*, 2nd ed., McGraw-Hill, N.Y., 1977.

Balke, B. Biodynamics: Human. In: *Medical Physics* (O. Glasser, ed) Chicago, Yearbook Publishers, 1960.

Bar-Or, O., and L.D. Zwiren. Maximal oxygen consumption test during arm exercise-reliability and validity. *J. Appl. Physiol.* 38:424-426, 1975.

Bonen, A., V.H. Heyward, K.J. Cureton, R.A. Borteau, and B.H. Massey. Prediction of maximal oxygen uptake in boys, ages 7-15 years. *Med. Sci. Sports*, 11:24-29, 1979.

Bonen, A., B.A. Wilson, M. Yarkony, and A.N. Belcastro. Maximal oxygen uptake during free, tethered and flume swimming. *J. Appl. Physiol.* 48:232-235, 1980.

Bouchard, C., P. Godbout, J.C. Mondor and C. Leblanc. Specificity of maximal aerobic power. *Eur. J. Appl. Physiol.*, 1979.

Carey, P., M. Stensland, and H.L. Hartley. Comparison of oxygen uptake during maximal work on the treadmill and rowing ergometer. *Med. Sci. Sports*. 6:101-103, 1974.

Costill, D.L. Metabolic responses during distance running. *J. Appl. Physiol.* 28:251-255, 1970.

Costill, D.L., J. Daniels, W. Evans, W. Fink, G. Krahenbul, B. Saltin: Skeletal Muscle Enzymes and Fiber Composition in Male and Female Track Athletes, *J. Appl. Physiol.* 40:149, 1976.

Costill, D.L., W.J. Fink, M.L. Pollock. Muscle fiber composition and enzyme activities of elite distance runners, *Med. Sci. Sports*. 8(2), 96, 1976.

Davies, C.T.M. Limitations to the prediction of maximum oxygen intake from cardiac frequency measurements. *J. Appl. Physiol.* 24:700-706, 1968.

Davis, J.A., P. Vodak, J.H. Wilmore, J. Vodak and P. Kurtz. Anaerobic threshold and maximal aerobic power for three modes of exercise. *J. Appl. Physiol.* 41:544-550, 1976.

Davis, J.A., M.H. Frank, B.J. Whipp and K. Wasserman: Anaerobic threshold alterations caused by endurance training in middle-aged men. *J. Appl. Physiol.: Respirat. Environ. Exercise Physiol.* 46:1039-1046, 1979.

Davis, H.A. and G.C. Gass. The anaerobic threshold as determined before and during lactic acidosis. *Eur. J. Appl. Physiol.* 47:141-149, 1981.

Ekblom, B., P.O. Åstrand, B. Saltin, J. Stenberg and B. Wallström. Effect of training on circulatory response to exercise. *J. Appl. Physiol.* 24:518-525, 1968.

Farrell, P.A., J.H. Wilmore, E.P. Coyle, J.E. Billing and D.L. Costill. Plasma lactate accumulation and distance running performance. *Med. Sci. Sports*. 11:338-344, 1979.

Ferguson, R.J., G.G. Marcotte, and R.R. Montpetit. Maximal oxygen uptake test during ice skating. *Med. Sci. Sports*. 1:207-211, 1969.

Fox, E. A simple, accurate technique for predicting maximal aerobic power. *J. Appl. Physiol.* 35:914-916, 1973.

Fox, E.L. *Sports Physiology*. W B Saunders, Toronto, 1979.

Gollnick, P.D., R.B. Armstrong, C.W. Saubert IV, K. Piehl, B. Saltin: Enzyme Activity and Fiber Composition in Skeletal Muscle of Trained and Untrained Men, *J. Appl. Physiol.*, 33:312, 1972.

Gollnick, P.D., L. Hermansen: Biochemical Adaptations to Exercise: Anaerobic Metabolism, *Exercise and Sports Sciences Reviews*, ed. J. Wilmore, Academic Press, Vol. 1:1, 1973.

Gollnick, P.D., K. Piehl, B. Saltin: Selective Glycogen Depletion Pattern in Human Muscle Fibers after Exercise of Varying Intensity and at Varying Pedalling Rates, *J. Physiol.*, 241:45, 1974.

Hagberg, J.M., M.D. Giese, and R.B. Schneider. Comparison of the three procedures for measuring VO_2 max in competitive cyclists. *Eur. J. Appl. Physiol.* 39:47-52, 1978.

Hagberg, J.M., E.F. Coyle, J.F. Miller, J.E. Carroll and W.H. Martin. Ventilatory threshold without increasing blood lactic acid levels in McArdle's Disease patients — anaerobic threshold? Abstract in *Med. Sci. Sports and Exercise*. 13: p.115, 1981.

Harrison, M.H., D.L. Bruce, G.A. Brown and L.A. Cochrane. A comparison of some indirect methods for predicting maximal oxygen uptake. *Aviat. Space Environ, Med.*, 51: 1128-33, 1980.

Hollman, W., T. Hettinger "Sportmedizin — Arbeits-und Traingsgrundlagen", F.K. Schatattauer Verlag, Stuttgart, 1976.

Jetté, M. A comparison between predicted VO_2 max from the Åstrand procedure and the Canadian Home Fitness Test. *Can. J. Appl. Sports. Sci.*, 4:214-218, 1979.

Kasch, F.W., W. Philips, J.E.L. Carter, J.L. Boyer. Cardiovascular Changes in Middle-aged Men During Two Hours of Training, *J. Appl. Physiol.*, 34:57-59, 1973.

Kasch, F.W., J.P. Wallace, R.R. Huhn, L.A. Krogh and P.M. Hurl. VO_2 max during horizontal and inclined treadmill running. *J. Appl. Physiol.* 40:982-983, 1976.

Katch, V., A. Weltman, S. Sody and P. Freedson, Validity of the relative percent concept for equating training intensity. *Eur. J. Appl. Physiol.* 39:219-227 (1978).

Keren, G., A. Magazanik and Y. Epstein. A comparison of various methods for the determination of VO_2 max. *Eur. J. Appl. Physiol.* 45:117-124, 1980.

Kindermann, W., G. Simon and J. Keul. The significance of the aerobic-anaerobic transition for the determination of work load intensities during endurance training. *European JAP*, 42:25-34, 1979.

Lange-Anderson, K., R.J. Shepard, H. Denolin, E. Varnauskas and R. Massironi. Fundamentals of exercise testing. *World Health Organization*, 1971.

MacDougall, J.D. The anaerobic threshold — its significance to the endurance athlete. *Can. J. Appl. Sports Sci.* 2:13-18, 1979.

Mathews, D.K., E.L. Fox. *The Physiological Basis of Physical Education and Athletics*. W.B. Saunders, Philadelphia, 1976.

McArdle, W., F. Katch and G. Pechar. Comparison of continuous and discontinuous treadmill and bicycle tests for max VO_2. *Med. Sci. Sports*, 5:156-160, 1973.

McLellan, T., T. Ferooh and J.S. Skinner. The effect of work load duration on the determination of the aerobic and anaerobic thresholds. Abstract in *Med. Sci. Sports and Exercise.* 13: p.69, 1981.

Montoye, H.J., R. Gayle. Familial relationships in maximal oxygen uptake. *Human Biology.* 50:241-249, 1978.

Pollock, M.L.: The Quantification of Endurance Training Programs. *Exercise and Sports Sciences Reviews*, ed. V.H. Wilmore, Academic Press Inc., Vol. 1:155, 1973.

Pugh, L.C.E. The influence of wind resistance in running and walking and the mechanical efficiency of work against horizontal or vertical forces. *J. Physiol.*, 213:255-276, 1971.

Roskamm, H., Optimum Patterns of Exercise for Healthy Adults, *Can. Med. Ass. J.*, 22:895, 1967.

Rowell, L.B.: Human Cardiovascular Adjustments to Exercise and Thermal Stress, *Physiol. Rev.*, 54:75, 1974.

Saltin, B., P.O. Åstrand, Maximal Oxygen Uptake in Athletes, *J. Appl. Physiol.*, 23:353, 1967.

Saltin, B., B. Blomquist, J.H. Mitchell, R.L. Johnson, Jr., K. Wildenthal, C.B. Chapman: Response to Submaximal and Maximal Exercise after Bed Rest and Training. *Circulation,* 38 (Suppl. 7): 1968.

Sjödin, B., I. Jacobs. Onset of blood lactate accumulation and marathon running performance. *Int. J. Sports Med.* 2:26-29, 1981.

Skinner, J.S. and T.H. McLellan. The transition from aerobic to anaerobic metabolism. *Res. Quart. for Ex. and Sport* 51:234-248, 1980.

Stamford, B.A. Step increment versus constant load tests for determination of maximal oxygen uptake. *Eur. J. Appl. Physiol.* 35:89-93, 1976.

Taylor, H.L., E. Buskirk and A. Henschal. Maximal oxygen intake as an objective measure of cardio-respiratory performance. *J. Appl. Physiol.* 8:73-80, 1955.

Wasserman, K., B.J. Whipp, S.N. Koyal and W.L. Beaver, Anaerobic threshold and respiratory gas exchange during exercise. *J. Appl. Physiol.* 35:236-243, 1973.

Wilson, B.A., A. Monego, M.K. Howard and M. Thompson. Specificity of maximal aerobic power measurement in trained runners. In *Science in Athletics* (eds. J. Terauds and G.G. Dales). Academic Pub. 213-217, 1979.

APPENDIX 4.1

Sample Consent Form

Treadmill Test For Measurement of Maximal Aerobic Power

The purpose of this test is to measure the maximal amount of oxygen which you can utilize while running. By measuring the amount of oxygen which you inhale and the amount of oxygen which you exhale, the amount which you utilize or consume can be calculated. This information can be used to assess the effectiveness of your past training as well as to help determine priorities for your future training program.

You will be given instructions on running on the treadmill and breathing through the collection system and be allowed to practise. After 5 or 6 minutes of warm-up, a technician will tape 3 electrodes to your chest for recording your heart rate. During the test you will run at ____ mph, and every 2 minutes the treadmill will be inclined upwards so that you will be running more and more uphill. We ask you to keep running until you feel that you are unable to maintain the pace set by the treadmill. At that point, grasp the safety rail, and the treadmill will be stopped.

Although you will be undergoing exercise to the point of temporary exhaustion, there is very little risk involved if you are a normal healthy individual. If you stumble or fall, the treadmill will be stopped immediately, and the consequences would be similar to if you had fallen on the track.

If blood sampling is to be performed (e.g., for lactic acid measurement), it will be done by a skilled technician. A hollow needle will be inserted into a peripheral vein in your arm and a small amount of blood (__ ml) will be drawn. There will be little discomfort associated with the procedure; there may, however, be slight bruising at the point of puncture.

Reporting of results.   It is understood that the results of this test will be reported only to:

☐   me

☐   my coach

☐   _____

I have read and understand the above explanation of the purpose and procedures for this test and agree to participate. I also understand that I am free to withdraw my consent at any time.

_____   _____
Signature   Witness

_____
Date

APPENDIX 4.2

Calculations of Oxygen Consumption

Required Data

1. Temperature of gas collected — usually in °C.

2. Volume of gas collected — if from a Tissot tank, this is usually the distance of deflection of the movable bell times the Tissot factor (liters of gas per cm of bell deflection).

3. The percentage of oxygen and carbon dioxide in both inspired and expired air.

Inspired oxygen and carbon dioxide must be determined in each laboratory. These values are fairly constant (i.e., 20.93% for O_2 and 0.03% CO_2 are used in our labs) but may differ slightly in different parts of the country.

Expired oxygen and carbon dioxide are determined by the gas analyzers from samples taken.

4. Frequency of respiration — counted during the collection of gas volume.

5. Barometric pressure — from a barometer (preferably of the mercury type) and used for calculating BTPS and STPD values.

Calculations

Basic Formula — for collection of gas on the expired side.

$$VO_2 \; \ell \cdot min^{-1} = (F_IO_2 \times V_I) - (F_EO_2 \times V_E)$$

where: F_EO_2 (fraction of expired O_2) =

$$\frac{\% \; O_2 \text{ in expired gas}}{100}$$

V_E (volume of air expired) =
determined from gas collection

F_IO_2 (fraction inspired O_2) =

$$\frac{\% \text{ of } O_2 \text{ in inspired gas (about 20.93)}}{100}$$

V_I (Volume of air inspired) =

$$\frac{V_E \times [100 - (\%O_2 \text{ expired} + \%CO_2 \text{ expired})]^*}{79.04}$$

*This corrects the expired volume by considering the difference in volume of O_2 uptake and CO_2 production. If these two values are equal, then $V_I = V_E$.

Both V_E and V_I are expressed in STPD (Stan-dard Temperature and Pressure, Dry) volumes when calculating VO_2. When calculating tidal volumes, and when comparing V (ventilation per minute), BTPS (Body Temperature and Pressure, Saturated) units often are used. Normally, the raw data units are collected as ATPS (Ambient Temperature and Pressure, Saturated) units. In this method of calculation, these factors may be calculated from the formula in Appendix 4.3. Alternatively, the ATPS to BTPS factor can be read from the table in Appendix 4.3 and the BTPS to STPD factor read from the table in Appendix 4.4. Values of pressure and temperature that do not appear on the tables can be interpolated. Note that the barometric pressure is indicated as being corrected. On mercury barometers with a brass scale, there is a correction factor for metal expansion at room temperature. Simply follow the directions accompanying the barometer used.

Example

Suppose gas is collected in a Tissot tank with a factor of 1.332 ℓ of gas for each 1 cm of deflection at a gas temperature in the Tissot of 21°C and a barometric pressure of 750 mm Hg.

The ATPS value would be: 1.332 × deflection in cm.

The BTPS value would be: ATPS value × 1.0971 (from Appendix 4.3 at 21°C and 750 mm Hg).

The STPD value would be: BTPS value × 0.8144 (from Appendix 4.4 at 750 mm Hg).

Other Calculated Data

Complete calculations normally include V_T (tidal volume), f (frequency of breathing) and R (respiratory exchange ratio). The V_T is simply the V_E (BTPS) divided by the f (respiratory frequency) as counted during the collection of gas. The respiratory exchange ratio is:

$$\frac{VCO_2 \text{ (volume of } CO_2 \text{ expired/min)}}{VO_2 \text{ (volume of } O_2 \text{ uptake/min)}}$$

and requires the VCO_2 to be calculated in the same way as VO_2. The basic formula is:

$$VCO_2 \; (\ell/min) = (F_ECO_2 \times V_E) - (F_ICO_2 \times V_I)$$

Normally, the F_ICO_2 is about 0.0003.

Therefore:

$$VCO_2 = (F_ECO_2 \times V_E) - (0.0003 \times V_I)$$

where:

$$F_ECO_2 = \frac{\% \text{ expired } CO_2}{100}$$

and V_I and V_E are in STPD units

VO_2 and VCO_2 values are expressed as liters per minute and may be expressed as $ml \cdot kg^{-1} \cdot min^{-1}$ by:

$$\frac{VO_2 \times 1000}{\text{body weight}}$$

Example of Calculations

Collected data:
Tissot factor = 1.332 ℓ/cm
Tissot temp. = 21.5°C
Corrected barometric pressure = 760 mm Hg
Body weight – 50.9 kg
Tissot deflection (30 s of collection) =
  52 cm × 2 = 104 cm for 60 s
%CO₂ in expired air = 3.90
%O₂ in expired air = 17.45
Breathing frequency = 66 breaths per minute
% inspired O₂ = 20.93

$$V_E \text{ ATPS} = 1.332 \times 104 = 138.53 \text{ ℓ/min}$$

$$V_E \text{ BTPS} = 1.0938 \times 138.53 = 151.52 \text{ ℓ/min}$$

$$V_E \text{ STPD} = 0.8258 \times 151.52 = 125.13 \text{ ℓ/min}$$

$$V_I \text{ STPD} = 125.13 \times \frac{[100 - (17.45 + 3.90)]}{79.04}$$

$$= 124.51 \text{ ℓ/min}$$

$$VO_2 \text{ STPD}, \text{ℓ/min} = (F_IO_2 \times V_I) - (F_EO_2 \times V_E)$$

$$= (0.2093 \times 124.51) - (0.1745 \times 125.13)$$

$$= 4.225$$

$$VCO_2 \text{ STPD}, \text{ℓ/min} = (F_ECO_2 \times V_E) - (0.0003 \times V_I)$$

$$= (0.0390 \times 125.13) - (0.0003 \times 124.51)$$

$$= 4.843$$

$$R = \frac{VCO_2}{VO_2}$$

$$= \frac{4.843}{4.225}$$

$$= 1.1463$$

$$V_T = \frac{V_E \text{ BTPS}}{f}$$

$$= \frac{151.52}{66}$$

$$= 2.296 \text{ ℓ}$$

and $$VO_2 \text{ ml} \cdot kg^{-1} \cdot min^{-1} = \frac{VO_2 \times 1000}{\text{wt.}}$$

$$= \frac{4225}{58.9}$$

$$= 71.73$$

APPENDIX 4.3

Conversion Factors for BTPS

$$\frac{273 + 37°C}{273 + \text{Temp. obs.}} \times \frac{\text{Bar. press.} - \text{pH}_2\text{O at temp. obs.}}{\text{Bar. press.} - \text{pH}_2\text{O at 37°C}}$$

Tissot Temp. (°C)	Corrected Bar. Press. (mm Hg)					
	730	740	750	760	770	780
19.0	1.1093	1.1086	1.1080	1.1073	1.1067	1.1061
19.5	1.1066	1.1059	1.1053	1.1046	1.1040	1.1034
20.0	1.1039	1.1032	1.1026	1.1019	1.1014	1.1008
20.5	1.1011	1.1005	1.0998	1.0992	1.0987	1.0981
21.0	1.0984	1.0978	1.0971	1.0965	1.0960	1.0954
21.5	1.0956	1.0950	1.0944	1.0938	1.0932	1.0927
22.0	1.0929	1.0923	1.0917	1.0911	1.0905	1.0900
22.5	1.0900	1.0895	1.0889	1.0883	1.0877	1.0872
23.0	1.0872	1.0867	1.0861	1.0856	1.0850	1.0845
23.5	1.0844	1.0838	1.0833	1.0828	1.0822	1.0817
24.0	1.0816	1.0810	1.0805	1.0800	1.0795	1.0790
24.5	1.0787	1.0781	1.0776	1.0772	1.0767	1.0762
25.0	1.0758	1.0753	1.0748	1.0744	1.0739	1.0734

APPENDIX 4.4

Factors for Changing BTPS Volumes To STPD Volumes

P_B	Correction Factor	P_B	Correction Factor	P_B	Correction Factor	P_B	Correction Factor	P_B	Correction Factor	P_B	Correction Factor
720	0.7796	729	0.7901	738	0.8005	747	0.8109	755	0.8201	763	0.8293
721	0.7808	730	0.7912	739	0.8017	748	0.8121	756	0.8212	764	0.8304
722	0.7820	731	0.7924	740	0.8028	749	0.8132	757	0.8224	765	0.8316
723	0.7831	732	0.7936	741	0.8040	750	0.8144	758	0.8235	766	0.8327
724	0.7843	733	0.7947	742	0.8051	751	0.8155	759	0.8247	767	0.8339
725	0.7854	734	0.7959	743	0.8063	752	0.8166	760	0.8258	768	0.8350
726	0.7866	735	0.7970	744	0.8075	753	0.8178	761	0.8270	769	0.8362
727	0.7878	736	0.7982	745	0.8086	754	0.8189	762	0.8281	770	0.8373
728	0.7889	737	0.7993	746	0.8098						

APPENDIX 4.5

Sample Computerized Reporting Form for Test Results
on Volleyball Players (University of Ottawa)

DATE: 810911   RANKING FOR VOLLEYBALL DATA, AUG 81

         ID.   : 4

VAR.   1.   SUBJECT'S NAME   :

Var. Number	Variable Name	Value		Rank	Percentile	Mean	# Cases
2.	Anaerobic pace (mph)	(9.5	)	2.00	87.5	9.94	8.
3.	Anaerobic duration (sec)	(30.6	)	7.00	25.0	65.61	8.
4.	Anaerobic lactate (mg%)	(103.2	)	5.00	50.0	96.66	8.
5.	Anaerobic hct (%)	(47.0	)	4.00	62.5	46.94	8.
6.	Jumping initial ht. (cm)	(225	)	7.00	25.0	232.25	8.
7.	Jumping / — ht. (cm)	(45	)	1.00	100.0	39.00	8.
8.	Jumping 1st trial HR	(144	)	5.00	50.0	145.50	8.
9.	Jumping final trial HR	(192	)	2.50	81.2	181.50	8.
10.	Jumping 5 min HR	(102	)	2.00	50.0	111.00	2.
11.	Jumping / — 91st jump (cm)	(7.0	)	1.00	100.0	1.00	7.
12.	Jumping / — 100th jump (cm)	(6.0	)	1.00	100.0	0.75	8.
13.	Jumping lactate (mg%)	(79.9	)	1.00	100.0	46.29	8.
14.	Jumping hct (%)	(46.5	)	3.00	75.0	45.88	8.
15.	Jumping he (gm%)	(15.7	)	4.00	62.5	15.60	8.
16.	Final speed (mph)	(8.0	)	4.50	56.2	8.00	8.
17.	Duration (min)	(8.0	)	4.00	62.5	7.56	8.
18.	MVO$_2$ speed (mph)	(8.0	)	4.50	56.2	8.00	8.
19.	MVO$_2$ (ml·kg^{-1}·min^{-1})	(47.3	)	6.00	37.5	49.39	8.
20.	V$_E$ STPD (ℓ·min^{-1})	(97.6	)	6.00	37.5	99.99	8.
21.	BF (bpm)	(42	)	1.00	100.0	42.00	1.
22.	VC ATPS (liters)	(3.94	)	7.50	18.7	4.56	8.
23.	Weight (kg)	(65.0	)	2.00	87.5	70.32	8.
24.	BV (wt.)	(61.68	)	2.00	87.5	67.11	8.
25.	Density (wt.)	(1.0722	)	5.00	50.0	1.07	8.
26.	% body fat	(10.51	)	4.00	62.5	12.04	8.
27.	Age (yrs.)	(22	)	5.50	43.7	22.00	8.
28.	Height (cm)	(170	)	8.00	12.5	177.63	8.

APPENDIX 4.6

Sample Computerized Reporting Form for Test Results on Volleyball Players (University of Ottawa)

DATE: 810911   RANKING FOR VOLLEYBALL DATA, AUG 81

Variable Number	Variable Name	Mean	# Cases
4.	ANAEROBIC LACTATE (MG%)	96.66	8.

		VALUE	RANK	PERCENTILE
ID: 1	Subject's name	(78.5)	2.00	87.5
ID: 2	Subject's name	(129.5)	8.00	12.5
ID: 3	Subject's name	(113.9)	7.00	25.0
ID: 4	Subject's name	(103.2)	5.00	50.0
ID: 5	Subject's name	(93.6)	4.00	62.5
ID: 6	Subject's name	(65.7)	1.00	100.0
ID: 7	Subject's name	(108.3)	6.00	37.5
ID: 8	Subject's name	(80.6)	3.00	75.0

Testing Maximal Anaerobic Power and Capacity

C. Bouchard • A.W. Taylor • S. Dulac

INTRODUCTION

The regeneration of muscle ATP through anaerobic mechanisms is an essential feature of sport performance. This area of exercise physiology and biochemistry has been characterized by dramatic advances over the past 50 years (Hill, Long, and Lupton, 1924; Margaria, Edwards, and Dill, 1933; Huckabee, 1958; Knuttgen, 1962). The development in the late sixties of the muscle biopsy technique as applied to physical work and performance has helped to clarify many of the mechanisms involved in anaerobic energy production.

Despite these advances and common acceptance by coaches and scientists that efforts of short duration and of maximum intensity are highly dependent upon anaerobic energy production mechanisms, there is little information available concerning the contribution of anaerobic metabolism to success in sport performances. Routine testing of the anaerobic energy production systems in athletes still is not a common feature of the sport science laboratories, and most sport scientists are not as well informed in this area as in some of the other areas of testing. Furthermore, the theoretical background and testing procedures are still undergoing rapid changes, thus preventing scientists from collecting sometimes relevant and useful data on athletes. The situation is, however, progressively changing, as this chapter will attempt to demonstrate.

Anaerobic Capacity vs. Anaerobic Power

As reviewed in Chapter 2, the energy sources for prolonged muscular exercise are lipid and carbohydrate (released through aerobic pathways) and for short-term intense exercise, glycogen and energy-rich phosphates (released through anaerobic pathways). The regeneration of ATP from ADP and CP does not result in the formation of lactic acid and is therefore termed *alactic*. The regeneration of ATP through the anaerobic breakdown of glycogen does result in the formation of lactic acid and is therefore termed *lactic*.

Table 5.1 Estimated maximal power and capacity of the three energy systems for a 70 kg reference man and a trained man[a] [b]

	MAXIMAL POWER ($kJ \cdot min^{-1}$)		MAXIMAL CAPACITY (kJ)	
	Average man	Trained man	Average man	Trained man
ATP $\twoheadrightarrow$ ADP + Pi CP $\twoheadrightarrow$ C + Pi	235-530	750	20-60	55
Glycogen $\twoheadrightarrow$ lactate	110-200	500	75-200	130-205
Glycogen FFA $\Big\}$ $\twoheadrightarrow$ CO_2 + H_2O	30-80	135-155	1,500-5,300	45,000-80,000

a) assuming: 20 kg of active muscle mass and 1 kcal = 4.2 kJ; 1 ℓ O_2 = 5 kcal = 21 kJ; 1 mole ATP = 42 kJ.
b) From Bouchard, Thibault, and Jobin (1981).

When assessing any of these energy systems, it is important to establish a distinction between the capacity and the power of the system. The total amount of energy available to perform work in a given energy system is referred to as the energetic *capacity* of that system. The maximal amount of energy that can be transformed during exercise, per units of time, is referred to as the energetic *power* of that system.

Table 5.1 constitutes a summary of data reported for the maximal power and capacity of each major energy system in untrained men as well as in trained athletes (Bouchard, Thibault, and Jobin, 1981). It can be observed that there are wide variations in estimated maximal values and that trained athletes tend to exhibit higher maximal anaerobic powers than untrained men. Although methodological differences, inherited genetic variations, assumptions with respect to body composition, and undoubtedly other influences may be contributing to these variations, it is generally believed by sport scientists that training is a significant causal factor. This is the rationale for monitoring in athletes their anaerobic capacities and powers during training.

Factors Affecting Anaerobic Power

Hermansen (1969) has hypothesized that the limiting factors for energy production and utilization for anaerobic work are as follows:

1. The rate of production of ATP in the muscle fiber.

2. The initial levels of muscle glycogen (Klausen, Piehl, and Saltin, 1975).

3. The ability to tolerate a high level of lactic acid: extremely high values of 25-26 $mM \cdot \ell^{-1}$ in the arterial blood and 20-30 $mM \cdot kg^{-1}$ muscle have been observed (Kinderman and Keul, 1977).

4. The ability to tolerate low intracellular pH: extreme values of 6.8 in the arterial blood and 6.4 in the muscle have been seen (Kinderman and Keul, 1977).

To these factors the following may be added:

5. The training level of the subjects: after training, Saltin and Karlsson (1971) observed, for a given power output, a decreased use of phosphagens and carbohydrate and a decreased production of lactic acid. Furthermore, the trained subjects were able to tolerate higher levels of both blood and muscle lactate.

6. The distribution of skeletal muscle fiber types, and the activities of the rate limiting enzymes in the various biochemical pathways may also be an important limitation for specific types of work related to the ST and FT fibers and the primarily used pathways (Taylor, 1980).

7. The efficiency of the cardiorespiratory system in transporting oxygen and of the oxygen utilization systems: the longer the bout of maximal work, the more critical this factor becomes. It is well established that oxygen consumption, heart rate, stroke volume, cardiac output, pulmonary ventilation, blood pressures, and other parameters increase rapidly during maximal work and reach almost a plateau in the first 2 to 3 min of exercise (Åstrand and Rodahl, 1970; Hollman, 1963).

A CONCEPTUAL FRAMEWORK

From a basic scientific point of view, it is useful to establish a distinction between the alactacid capacity, the alactacid power, the lactacid capacity, and the lactacid power of the anaerobic energy production system. This could then be translated into a four-component system that theoretically might be used to test in an orderly manner the anaerobic energy characteristics of athletes. Metabolic events associated with anaerobic performance suggest the following time frame for each of these components.

1. Alactacid anaerobic capacity: total energy output during a maximal effort lasting 10 to 15 s.

2. Alactacid anaerobic power: maximum rate (e.g., per second) of energy output during a maximal effort lasting 10 to 15 s.

3. Lactacid anaerobic capacity: total energy output during a maximal effort lasting from about 60 to 120 s.

4. Lactacid anaerobic power: maximum rate of energy output during a maximal effort highly saturated in glycolytic energy production. The actual period of measurement would vary with the total duration of the work test.

Relevance

The laboratory measurements of anaerobic performance are obviously of relevance only to those athletes whose sport requires a significant contribution from one (or both) of the alactic and lactic pathways. It would therefore be of greatest relevance to athletes of most team sports and to those athletes who require maximum power output over a time ranging from approximately 5 s to 6 min (see Table 4.2 in Chapter 4). Performance in events of shorter duration (e.g., jumping or throwing) or of longer duration (e.g., 10,000 m in track) will be influenced primarily by factors other than anaerobic energy potential.

As is the case in testing maximal aerobic power (Chapter 4), laboratory tests of maximal anaerobic power and capacity are of greatest relevance to the athlete when they simulate his actual mode of exercise and involve the specific muscle groups which he uses in his sport. For many sports, this means that commercially available ergometry equipment will have to be modified, while for others, specific equipment will have to be constructed. For still others, anaerobic power and capacity testing can probably be conducted best in the field setting (see Chapter 8).

RECOMMENDED TESTING PROCEDURES

When testing the anaerobic energy production characteristics of athletes, it seems appropriate to consider separately the alactic and the lactic work outputs. For practical purposes, two types of tests are recommended:

1. *A test of alactic anaerobic capacity.*

This would involve a maximal effort lasting for approximately 10 to 15 s in order to obtain the maximum energy output under predominantly anaerobic alactacid conditions. The results of such a test would also provide an index of maximal alactic anaerobic power.

2. *A test of lactacid anaerobic capacity.*

This would involve a maximal effort lasting for approximately 60 to 90 s in order to obtain the maximum energy output under predominantly anaerobic lactic conditions. Although several factors may contribute to fatigue under such conditions (and therefore affect total power output), the major factor may be assumed to be the ability to tolerate a lower intracellular pH.

Measurements of each of these two anaerobic characteristics can best be achieved by computing either the amount of mechanical work that can be done in a specified time, or by monitoring the time required to perform a given amount of presumably anaerobic work. The latter will be generally less preferable and less precise than the former. Valid and reliable measurements of anaerobic capacity can be made only when appropriate ergometer devices are available. Tests could be carried out easily, with varying degrees of sophistication, on a leg cycle ergometer, an arm cranking

ergometer, a rowing ergometer, a paddling ergometer, etc., and with more isolated muscle groups, in controlled and specific movement patterns designed to fit the needs of the athletes.

To answer additional questions related to the status of the athlete's anaerobic capacities and powers, the sport scientist may sometimes want to obtain measurements of oxygen debt, or of other physiological and metabolic indicators in the blood or in the skeletal muscle, during work or in the recovery period. One must keep in mind, however, that these parameters are not direct measurements of anaerobic capacities or powers, but, rather, reflect conditions under which measurements were performed.

EXISTING LABORATORY AND FIELD TESTS

The authors of this chapter have collected several anaerobic laboratory and field tests from the literature. There are obvious limitations to this brief survey; much more has been attempted than has been reported in the literature available to the authors. It is the purpose of this section to present a brief description of each of these tests, along with indications of the reliability of the procedures and the availability of norms. Moreover, indications as to how these tests were used with different populations are introduced. Although a concise description of procedures is submitted for each test, the sport scientist should get the original reports in order to obtain a more complete outline before embarking on the systematic use of any of these tests.

We have attempted to specify the aim of each test in terms of alactic capacity or alactic power, lactic capacity or lactic power. As a result, this terminology will seldom be found as such in the literature. Hopefully, this will not detract significantly from the original intentions of the test designers and will give the reader a better understanding of the proposed system.

The sport scientist faced with the evaluation of anaerobic capacities and powers of athletes must give some thought to the most appropriate ways of expressing results. Indications about this issue are rather scarce in the literature. One finds anaerobic capacities and powers expressed in absolute values, per kilogram of body weight, per square meter of BSA, per kilogram of LBM, per unit of limb muscle mass, and others. The sport scientist should explore in each case, with both the coach and the athlete, which procedure is more meaningful and more discriminating.

Margaria, Aghemo, and Rovelli Test (1966)

Aim of the test:
Measurement of alactacid anaerobic power.

Exercise and procedures:
Staircase (stair: 175 mm high); 2 switchmats connected to a time recorder (sensitivity: 0.01 s). The subject is asked to run at top speed, two steps at a time, up a staircase. A switchmat is placed on the 8th and 12th stair (4th and 6th step).

Results:

$$P = \frac{W \times 9.8 \times D}{T}$$

P: alactacid power (watt)
9.8: normal acceleration of gravity in $m \cdot sec^{-2}$

W: weight of the subject (kg)
D: vertical height between first and second switchmat (m)
T: time from first to second switchmat (s)

There are no norms as such, but selected data reported thus far are presented in Table 5.2.

Reliability:
Within a testing session: 4% variation
2 subjects measured several times within a 5 week period: 2% variation
Test-retest: 0.85

Margaria-Kalamen Power Test (Kalamen, 1968)

Aim of the test:
Measurement of alactic anaerobic power.

Exercise and procedures:
Staircase (stair: 174 mm high); 2 switchmats

Table 5.2   Published data for the Margaria, Aghemo, and Rovelli (1966) anaerobic power test

| | ANAEROBIC ALACTACID POWER | | |
POPULATION	Watts	Watts/kg	REFERENCE
Untrained men	1211.1	16.7	Thompson, Andrew and Garvie (1980)
Marathoners	948.3	14.7	Thompson, Andrew and Garvie (1980)
Sprinters	1246.4	17.7	Thompson, Andrew and Garvie (1980)
Football players:			
Ends	1164.3	13.9	Costill et al. (1968)
Blockers	1464.0	13.7	Costill et al. (1968)
Guards	1387.3	14.6	Costill et al. (1968)
Backfielders	1257.5	15.0	Costill et al. (1968)
Orienteering runners:			
Male	1006.2	13.9	Knowlton et al. (1980)
Female	751.2	13.0	Knowlton et al. (1980)
Hockey players:			
Forwards	1367.0	17.7	Green and Houston (1975)
Defensemen	1403.3	17.3	Green and Houston (1975)
Goalkeepers	1049.3	14.3	Green and Houston (1975)
Olympic athletes:			
Pentathletes		18.9	Di Prampero et al, (1970)
Wrestlers		17.2	Di Prampero et al. (1970)
Runners: long distance			
middle distance		16.7	Di Prampero et al. (1970)
sprint			
Soccer players, boxers, fencers		15.0	Di Prampero et al. (1970)
Shooters		14.1	Di Prampero et al. (1970)
Rowers		13.7	Di Prampero et al. (1970)
Swimmers, field hockey players		11.5	Di Prampero et al. (1970)
Men 20-29 years		15.2	Margaria et al. (1966)
Sprinters		27.5	Margaria et al. (1966)
Middle distance runners		20.2	Margaria et al. (1966)
P.E. Students men		15.2	Sawka et al. (1980)
P.E. Students women		12.3	Sawka et al. (1980)

connected to a time recorder (sensitivity: 0.01 s). The subject stands 6 m in front of the staircase. Subject runs up the stairs as rapidly as possible, taking 3 steps at a time. A switchmat is placed on the 3rd and 6th stair.

Results:

$$P = \frac{W \times 9.8 \times D}{T}$$

P: alactacid power (watt)
9.8: normal acceleration of gravity in $m \cdot sec^{-2}$
W: weight of the subject (kg)
D: vertical height between first and second switchmat (m)
T: time from 1st to 2nd switchmat (s)

Table 5.3 and Table 5.4 present norms and data published on athletes.

Reliability:
Not reported.

Wingate Anaerobic Power Test (1977)

Aim of the test:
Measurement of alactacid anaerobic capacity and lactacid capacity.

Exercise and procedures:
Bicycle ergometer for the leg test; adapted bicycle ergometer for the arm test; electrically triggered counter. Warm-up allowed with a target heart rate of 150 bpm.

Work load:
Leg test: children (<15 years): 35 g/kg body

Table 5.3   Published norms for the Margaria-Kalamen alactacid anaerobic power test (Kalamen, 1968)

| CLASSIFICATION | MEN: AGE GROUPS IN YEARS | | | | |
	15-20	20-30	30-40	40-50	50
Poor	<1113[a]	<1044	< 838	< 642	< 495
Below average	1114-1466	1045-1368	839-1093	643-828	496-642
Average	1467-1839	1369-1721	1094-1377	829-1034	643-809
Good	1840-2197	1722-2059	1378-1647	1035-1225	810-961
Excellent	>2197	>2059	>1647	>1225	> 961

| CLASSIFICATION | WOMEN: AGE GROUPS IN YEARS | | | | |
	15-20	20-30	30-40	40-50	50
Poor	< 907	< 834	< 642	< 495	< 378
Below average	908-1181	835-1093	643-828	496-642	379-475
Average	1182-1485	1094-1378	829-1034	643-809	476-603
Good	1486-1785	1379-1648	1035-1226	810-961	604-735
Excellent	>1785	>1648	>1226	> 961	> 735

a) Values in watts.

Table 5.4   Data reported in athletes for the Margaria-Kalamen anaerobic test

| SUBJECTS | ALACTACID ANAEROBIC POWER | | |
	Watts	Watts/kg	REFERENCE
Alpine skiers:			
male	1791	23.7	Haymes and Dickinson (1980)
female	1131	19.2	Haymes and Dickinson (1980)
Cross-country skiers:			
male	1534	21.0	Haymes and Dickinson (1980)
female	989	17.7	Haymes and Dickinson (1980)
Nordic combined	1470	20.9	Haymes and Dickinson (1980)

weight; adults: 45 g/kg body weight for a Fleisch ergometer; for a Monark ergometer, the resistance would be 75 g/kg body weight for adults.

Arm test: 50 g/kg body weight for Monark ergometer; 30 g/kg body weight for Fleisch ergometer.

Duration of exercise: 30 s.

The subject is instructed to pedal as fast as possible for 30 s. The resistance is adjusted in the first 2 or 3 s and at that time, the clock and the electronic counter are activated. The number of pedal revolutions is recorded every 5 s.

Results:

Alactacid capacity: maximal power observed in a 5 s period (watt or watt/kg body weight).

Lactacid capacity: total work performed in 30 s (joules or joules/kg body weight).

Table 5.5 contains some of the data reported thus far for the Wingate anaerobic test.

Reliability:

0.90 to 0.93 (test-retest at 1 or 2 weeks interval).
0.95 to 0.98 (test-retest on same day).

De Bruyn-Prévost Test (1974)

Aim of the test:

Measurement of lactacid anaerobic capacity.

Exercise and procedures:

Bicycle ergometer; metronome.
Workload in males: 400 W
Workload in females: 350 W
Pedal rhythm for males: 124-128 rpm
Pedal rhythm for females: 104-108 rpm
In the first 5 s, the workload is increased from 50 to 400 W for men and 50 to 350 W for women.

End of the test: when the subject is not able to maintain the required pedal rhythm.

Results:

Delay time: time required to reach the required pedal rhythm.

Total time: total duration up to the end of the test.

$$\text{Index: } \frac{\text{total time}}{\text{delay time}}$$

The index and the blood lactate are used to evaluate lactacid tolerance.

Table 5.6 introduces some of the results published with the present test.

Reliability:

Test-retest: 0.77.

Table 5.5　A review of selected data reported for the Wingate anaerobic test

POPULATION	ALACTACID CAPACITY		LACTACID CAPACITY		REFERENCE
	Watts	Watts/kg	Joules	Joules/kg	
Cross-country runners: 10 years old			4766	149.4	Mayers and Gutin (1979)
10 year old controls			3883	119.9	Mayers and Gutin (1979)
Swimmers: leg test — competitive			5780	182.9	Inbar and Bar-Or (1977)
— recreation			5464	182.1	Inbar and Bar-Or (1977)
Swimmers: arm test — competitive			3481	110.2	Inbar and Bar-Or (1977)
— recreation			3067	102.2	Inbar and Bar-Or (1977)
7- 9 year old boys	159.8	5.88	4463	164	Inbar and Bar-Or (1975)
11-12 year old boys	322		8135		Grodjinovsky et al. (1980)
19-21 year old men — legs			17686		Ayalon, Inbar, and Bar-Or (1974)
— arms			9091		Ayalon, Inbar, and Bar-Or (1974)
Junior synchronized swimmers			9051	182.4	Poole, Crépin, and Sévigny (1980)
Senior synchronized swimmers			10674	187.8	Poole, Crépin, and Sévigny (1980)
Israëli males:　9-10 years				171.6	Bar-Or, Dotan, and Inbar (1977)
10-11 years				186.3	Bar-Or, Dotan, and Inbar (1977)
11-12 years				183.9	Bar-Or, Dotan, and Inbar (1977)
13-14 years				213.3	Bar-Or, Dotan, and Inbar (1977)
19-22 years				213.3	Bar-Or, Dotan, and Inbar (1977)
30-40 years				210.8	Bar-Or, Dotan, and Inbar (1977)
Male sprinters, jumpers				255-314	Bar-Or, Dotan, and Inbar (1977)
Israëli females: 10-11 years				166.7	Bar-Or, Dotan, and Inbar (1977)
13-14 years				176.5	Bar-Or, Dotan, and Inbar (1977)
30-40 years				171.6	Bar-Or, Dotan, and Inbar (1977)
Female hurdlers				281.9	Bar-Or, Dotan, and Inbar (1977)

Table 5.6   A review of data published for the De Bruyn-Prévost lactacid anaerobic capacity test

POPULATION	DELAY (S)	DURATION OF TEST (S)	INDEX	LACTIC ACID (MG %)	REFERENCE
Young adult males	11.0	46.0	4.58	115.0	De Bruyn-Prévost (1974)
Young adult females	11.6	38.5	3.50	76.5	Heyters and Poortmans (1977)
Young adult males	4.8	51.3	11.30		Heyters and Poortmans (1977)
P.E. students, males	10.6	44.9	4.80	97.0	De Bruyn-Prévost (1980)
P.E. students, females	11.1	42.5	4.30	79.3	De Bruyn-Prévost (1980)

Table 5.7   A review of data published for the Katch anaerobic test

POPULATION	ALACTACID CAPACITY		LACTACID CAPACITY		REFERENCE
	Watts	Watts/kg	Joules	Joules/kg	
Young adult males	564	7.4	51,602	676	Katch (1974)
Young adult males	677	9.5	42,929	603	Katch and Weltman (1979)

Katch Test (Katch, 1974, and Katch and Weltman, 1979)

Aim of the test:
Measurement of alactacid capacity and lactacid capacity.

Exercise and procedures:
Monark bicycle ergometer and electrically-triggered counter.
Workload: 34 kp/rev or 5.6 kp on the ergometer scale.
Duration: 120 s.
At the signal, the subject pedals as fast as possible and the workload is adjusted within 1.5 s.
Subject is not informed as to the exact length of the test, except that it is very short.
Subject is asked to do as many revolutions as possible, with strong verbal encouragements.
Subject is not allowed to lift off the seat.

Results:
Lactacid capacity: total work produced during the test.
Alactacid anaerobic capacity: maximal work output during first 6 s.
Table 5.7 introduces some of the data published for the Katch test.

Reliability:
Lactacid anaerobic capacity test-retest: 0.92.

The Lactacid Tolerance Test of Szögÿ and Cherebetiu (1974)

Aim of the test:
Measurement of lactacid anaerobic capacity.

Exercise and procedures:
The test is performed on the bicycle ergometer. Subject must accomplish as much work as possible in 1 min. Work load is adjusted for body weight and remains constant during the test. The number of revolutions is counted and total amount of work computed.

Results:
Expressed in total amount of kpm during 1 min. Data reported for athletes in the original paper have been estimated from graphs and are reported in Table 5.8.

Reliability:
None reported.

Anaerobic Treadmill Test of Cunningham and Faulkner (1969)

Aim of the test:
Measurement of lactacid anaerobic capacity.

Exercise and procedures:
Motor-driven treadmill.
Treadmill grade: 20%.

Adults: 7 or 8 mph (time to exhaustion: between 30 and 60 s).

Children: 134, 188, and 214 m/s for 10, 15, and 21 years (time to exhaustion: between 45 and 90 s).

Results:

Running time in s.

O_2 debt: measured over a 12 min period after exercise.

Blood lactate: 5 and 12 min post-exercise.

Some of the data reported for the Cunningham and Faulker anaerobic test are presented in Table 5.9.

Reliability:

Running time: 0.76 to 0.91.

O_2 debt: 0.62 to 0.96.

Blood lactate: 0.49 to 0.79.

Marrin, Sharratt, and Taylor Treadmill Test (1980)

Aim of the test:

Measurement of lactacid anaerobic capacity.

Exercise and procedures:

Running on a motor-driven treadmill: 20%

Table 5.8   Data submitted for a 1 min bicycle ergometer lactacid capacity test by Szögÿ and Cherebetiu (1974)

ATHLETES	KPM/MIN[a]	BODY WEIGHT IN KG	JOULES/KG
Professional cycling (9)[b]	3240	72.7	713.2
Weight lifting (11)	3100	86.8	851.5
Volleyball (24)	3060	82.1	805.4
Biathlon (9)	3050	70.2	688.7
Cycling (road) (16)	3040	69.8	684.7
European handball (20)	3020	80.4	788.7
Waterpolo (17)	2980	81.1	795.6
Speed ice skating (9)	2950	68.7	673.9
Kayak (18)	2880	79.1	776.0
Sprinting (9)	2760	75.8	743.6
Wrestling (Greco-Roman) (13)	2740	78.7	772.1
Wrestling (freestyle) (22)	2700	74.1	726.9
Soccer (26)	2650	72.4	710.2
Canoe (10)	2580	75.4	739.7
Boxing (25)	2450	70.1	687.7

a) Estimated from graph.
b) In parentheses, number of athletes.

---

grade, 8 mph.

Run as long as possible, 4 min rest, and run as long as possible.

Results:

Sum of the 2 running times.

Blood lactate: 5 and 10 min post-exercise.

The test was designed to be used with wrestlers. Preliminary norms have been proposed by the authors and are reported in Table 5.10.

Reliability:

None reported thus far.

Jetté, Thoden, and Reed Anaerobic Capacity Test (1975)

Aim of the test:

Measurement of lactacid anaerobic capacity.

Exercise and procedures:

The test is performed on a Quinton bicycle ergometer with a pedal rhythm of 90 rpm.

Initial workload of 300 kpm/min followed by an increase of 200 kpm/min every 5 s up to a maximum workload of 2400 kpm/min.

The test is ended when the subject is not able to maintain the required pedal rhythm.

Results:

Measurement of VO_2 during the test.

Blood lactate before, and 5 min post, test.

Reliability:

None seems to have been reported.

A Bicycle Test of Alactacid Anaerobic Capacity (Simoneau et al., submitted)

Aim of the test:

Measurement of alactacid anaerobic capacity.

Exercise and procedures:

This test is performed on a modified Monark ergocycle. A photoelectric cell registers each third of a flywheel revolution and relays the data to a micro-processor. A potentiometer connected to the tension adjustment mechanism of the ergocycle registers the work load. An electrical timing system controls the input to the micro-processor, and the total work performed each second is computed. Initial workload is determined according to body weight (about 0.09 kp/kg), but it is manually adjusted during the test so that the subject can maintain a high pedalling speed of 10 to 16 m/s.

Table 5.9 A summary of data published for the anaerobic test of Cunningham and Faulkner

POPULATION	RUNNING TIME (s)	O₂ DEBT (ℓ)	BLOOD LACTATE	REFERENCE
Males 23-41 years old:				
pre-training	52	6.63	101 mg %	Cunningham and Faulkner (1969)
post-training	64	7.26	118 mg %	Cunningham and Faulkner (1969)
Competitive ice hockey players:				
10 years old		2.05	80.0 mM/ℓ	Paterson, Cunningham, and Bonk (1980)
15 years old		5.29	12.0 mM/ℓ	Paterson, Cunningham, and Bonk (1980)
21 years old		7.90	15.1 mM/ℓ	Paterson, Cunningham, and Bonk (1980)
Junior ice hockey players:				
forwards pre-season	66		104 mg %	Green and Houston (1975)
post-season	75		118 mg %	Green and Houston (1975)
defensemen pre-season	60		115 mg %	Green and Houston (1975)
post-season	74		125 mg %	Green and Houston (1975)

The test itself consists of two 10 s all-out trials. The following directions are given to the subject:

1. Always pedal in a seated position.

2. At the first signal, pedal at 80 rpm (while the work load is rapidly adjusted — within 2-3 s — by the investigator).

3. At the command "start," pedal as fast as possible during 10 s. (Strong verbal encouragements are given throughout the test).

After the first trial and a 10 min resting period, a second trial is executed.

Results:

Work output in joules (J) or in joules/kg of body weight (J/kg) during the best 10 s performance.

Table 5.11 describes some of the data reported by Simoneau et al.

Table 5.10 Preliminary norms reported for the lactacid anaerobic capacity treadmill test of Marrin, Sharratt, and Taylor

RUNNING TIME IN S	EVALUATION	LACTIC ACID (mg % over resting level)
<30	not acceptable	
30-40	poor	
40-50	fair	80
50-60	average	90
60-70	good	100
70-80	very good	120
>80	excellent	150

Reliability:

Intra-class coefficient of 0.98.

A Bicycle Test of Lactacid Anaerobic Capacity (Simoneau et al., submitted)

Aim of the test:

Measurement of lactacid anaerobic capacity.

Exercise and procedures:

The test is performed on a modified Monark ergocycle (see description of previous test).

The workload is determined according to body weight (about 0.05 kp/kg), but it is manually adjusted during the test to maintain a speed between 10 and 16 m/s.

The test consists of a 90 s all-out ergocycle performance. The subject has to —

1. pedal in a seated position;

2. pedal at 80 rpm at the first signal while the workload is rapidly adjusted (within 2-3 s) by the investigator;

3. at the command "start," pedal at approximately 130 rpm for the first 20 s, and as fast as possible after this time. Strong verbal encouragements are given throughout the test.

Results:

Lactacid anaerobic capacity is expressed as the total work output in joules (J) or in joules/kg of body weight (J/kg) during the 90 s performance.

Data reported by Simoneau et al. for this test are presented in Table 5.11.

Reliability:

Intra-class coefficient of 0.99.

A Side-Step Test of Anaerobic Capacity
(Song, 1982)

Aim of the test:
Measurement of lactacid capacity.

Exercise and procedure:
Subject stands at a center line; jumps 30 cm to the right (left) and touches the line; jumps back to the center; jumps to the left (right) and touches the line; jumps back to the center; as fast and as many times as possible for 1 min. One complete cycle will be recorded as 1 and half a cycle as 0.5.

Results:
Expressed in total number of repetitions during 1 min.

Reliability:
0.92.

TENTATIVE NORMS				
Poor	Fair	Average	Good	High
		Female		
<33	34-37	38-41	42-45	46+
		Male		
<37	38-41	42-45	46-49	50+

Table 5.11   Data reported for the bicycle anaerobic tests described by Simoneau et al.

	ANAEROBIC ALACTACID CAPACITY		ANAEROBIC LACTACID CAPACITY	
	Joules (SD)	Joules/kg (SD)	Joules (SD)	Joules/kg (SD)
Young males	6,849 (1,982)	108 (16)	34,218 (4,137)	486 (50)
Young females	5,128 (1,020)	90 (14)	22,280 (2,463)	377 (34)

Table 5.12   Norms for the lactacid anaerobic capacity ice skating test of Larivière and Godbout (1976)
(twelve times 60 ft.; units in seconds)

	CATEGORIES				
PERCENTILE	Novice	Mosquito	Pee-Wee	Bantam	Midget
100	45.4	50.7	47.1	44.5	44.3
95	61.6	57.5	54.8	48.8	48.0
90	63.4	58.5	55.6	50.3	48.8
85	63.8	59.4	56.5	51.6	49.0
80	64.3	60.1	57.3	52.8	49.6
75	65.5	61.1	57.9	53.4	50.0
70	66.3	61.4	58.3	54.0	50.5
65	66.9	61.9	59.0	54.5	51.0
60	67.8	62.3	59.6	55.0	51.2
55	68.0	62.8	60.0	55.2	51.5
50	68.5	63.5	60.9	56.0	51.7
45	68.9	63.8	61.3	56.3	52.1
40	70.0	64.4	61.7	57.0	52.3
35	71.0	65.2	62.0	57.6	52.6
30	72.0	66.0	62.7	58.0	53.0
25	73.1	66.9	63.5	58.8	54.5
20	74.2	67.9	64.5	59.6	54.9
15	74.8	69.1	65.7	60.4	55.5
10	78.7	71.3	67.2	61.6	56.6
5	88.5	74.4	71.0	65.0	57.9
0	96.8	77.9	75.9	68.5	59.9
N cases	67	285	249	102	93
Mean	71.1	64.3	61.5	56.4	52.2
SD	10.0	5.3	5.6	4.7	3.0

The Basketball Anaerobic Field Test of Burke (1980)

The test is described in Figure 5.1. Little has been reported about this test. It has been indicated that performance of guards in this test ranges from 25 to 27 s, while performance of other players reaches about 29 to 31 s.

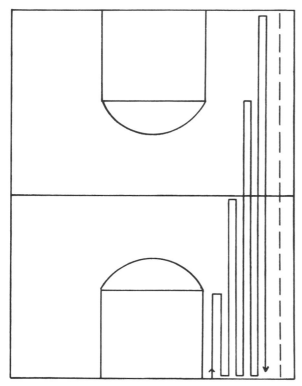

Fig. 5.1   A test of anaerobic power for basketball. The drill is run in a straight line. (From Burke, 1980).

A Running Test of Anaerobic Capacity (Thomson, 1981)

Subject must sprint around a 400 m track. The cumulative time for any distance beyond 200 m is well correlated ($r = -.74$) with a laboratory measurement of anaerobic capacity. The best prediction of laboratory anaerobic capacity relied upon two parameters:

— time (s) to 256 m: a
— speed in m/min between 256 and 329 m: b.
The following prediction equation ($R = 0.82$;

$p < 0.01$) was suggested by the author.
Anaerobic capacity (kcal/kg) =
$1.72 - (0.027 \times a + 0.022 \times b)$

Anaerobic Ice Skating Tests for Hockey Players

Anaerobic Alactacid Capacity Test (Jetté, Thoden, and Reed, 1975)

Subject skates as fast as possible from one goal line to the other (180 ft.).
A reliability of 0.77 has been reported.

The Lactacid Anaerobic Capacity Test of Larivière and Godbout (1976)

Subject must skate as fast as possible twelve times 60 ft., i.e., 6 times back and forth, with quick stops and starts. The time of the performance is reported in seconds. In a test-retest reliability study, a correlation of 0.96 was reported by the authors. Authors also have published norms for various age groups of young ice hockey players. These percentile norms are reproduced in Table 5.12.

CONDUCTING THE TESTS

Personnel

Tests must be conducted by trained and qualified technicians or investigators. Results of these tests, because of their inherent complexities, must be interpreted by competent sport scientists.

Safety Measures

Proper security measures associated with any work tests must be employed whenever anaerobic tests are performed in the laboratory. Additional and special precautions should be taken to avoid falls resulting from dizziness associated with sudden cessation of work after a brief maximal period of exercise. A strict criterion for rapid cessation of the test must be used and applied for subjects where excess security is warranted.

Equipment

Most of the anaerobic tests require a precise measure of mechanical work performed over a short period of time, or a precise measurement of elapsed time. Equipment must therefore be precisely and regularly calibrated.

Preparation of Subjects

Subjects should be dressed for a maximal exercise test. Subjects must be allowed to become familiar with the kind of exercise to be performed. In general, they should be allowed to warm up prior to the test; for some of the tests reported in this chapter, however, it has been suggested that no warm-up be permitted before the test. The investigator must therefore be aware that procedures may sometimes deviate slightly from the original work. Verbal encouragement should be given to subjects during the test.

In brief, procedures should be standardized with respect to explanations about the test, warm-up, simulation of tests, and encouragement during the test itself.

Reporting of Results

Results of all anaerobic power tests should be reported in international units of measurements (see Chapter 3). At the present time, comparisons between tests are complex because different units of measurements and procedures are used. Thus, whenever possible, measurements of lactacid capacity should be expressed in joules (J) or kilojoules (kJ), whereas measurements of anaerobic power ought to be reported in joules or kilojoules per minute, or in watts.

In all cases, absolute measurements as well as scores per kilogram of body weight should be the minimum reported and interpreted to coaches and athletes.

Summary

At the present time, valid and reliable tests of anaerobic capacities and powers can be conducted on a bicycle ergometer. Some of the components can be obtained with running on the treadmill, or on the track, or with ice skating. Much remains to be done in order to provide valid and reliable testing systems which could satisfy the requirement of sport specificity. Furthermore, establishment of norms for sport applications in this area has yet to be undertaken.

REFERENCES

Åstrand, P.O. and K. Rodahl. *Textbook of Work Physiology.* New York, McGraw-Hill, 1970.

Ayalon, A., O. Inbar and O. Bar-Or. Relationships among measurements of explosive strength and anaerobic power. In: *International Series on Sports Sciences, Vol. 1, Biomechanics IV. Proceedings of the Fourth International Seminar on Biomechanics.* R.C. Nelson and C.A. Morehouse (eds). Baltimore, University Park Press, 1975, pp. 572-577.

Bar-Or, O., R. Dotan and O. Inbar. A 30 sec. all-out ergometric test — its reliability and validity for anaerobic capacity. *Israël J. Med. Sci.* 13: 126, 1977.

Bouchard, C., M.C. Thibault and J. Jobin. Advances in human work physiology. *Yearbook of Physical Anthropology.* 24: 1-36, 1981.

Burke, E.J. Physiological considerations and suggestions for the training of elite basketball players. in: *Toward an understanding of human performance.* E.J. Burke (ed). Ithaca, Movement Publications, 1980, pp. 293-311.

Costill, D.L., W.M. Hoffman, F. Kehoe, S.J. Miller and W.C. Myers. Maximum anaerobic power among college football players. *J. Sports Med. Phys. Fitness,* 8: 103-106, 1968.

Cunningham, D.A. and J.A. Faulkner. The effect of training on aerobic and anaerobic metabolism during a short exhaustive run. *Med. Sci. Sports,* 1: 65-69, 1969.

De Bruyn-Prévost, P. A short anaerobic physical fitness test on the bicycle ergometer. *Proceedings of the Third European Congress of Sports Medicine.* Budapest, Hungary, 1974.

De Bruyn-Prévost, P. Determination of anaerobic physical fitness (anaerobic endurance). In: *Kinanthropometry II. International series on sport sciences.* M. Ostyn, G. Beunen and J. Simons (eds). Baltimore, University Park Press, 1980, pp. 481-488.

Di Prampero, P.E., F. Pinera Limas and G. Sassis. Maximal muscular power, aerobic and anaerobic, in 116 athletes performing at the XIXth Olympic Games in Mexico. *Ergonomics,* 13: 665-674, 1970.

Edwards, R.H.T., N.L. Jones, E.A. Oppenheimer, R.L. Hughes and R.P. Knill-Jones. Interrelation of responses during progressive exercise in trained and untrained subjects. *Quart. J. Exp. Physiol.,* 54: 394-403, 1969.

Fox, E.L. *Sports Physiology,* Philadelphia, Saunders, 1979.

Gollnick, P.D., K. Piehl, J. Karlsson and B. Saltin. Glycogen depletion patterns in human skeletal muscle fibers after varying types and intensities of exercise. In: *Metabolic adaptation to prolonged physical exercise.* H. Howald and J.R. Poortmans (eds.). Basel, Birkhäuser, 1975, pp. 416-421.

Green, H.J. and M.E. Houston. Effect of a season of ice hockey on energy capacities and associated functions. *Med. Sci. Sports,* 7: 299-303, 1975.

Grodjinovsky, A., O. Inbar, R. Dotan and O. Bar-Or. Training effect on the anaerobic performance of children as measured by the Wingate anaerobic test. In: *Children and exercise IX.* K. Berg and B.O. Eriksson (eds). Baltimore, University Park Press. 1980, pp. 139-145.

Haymes, E.M. and A.L. Dickinson. Characteristics of elite male and female ski racers. *Med. Sci. Sports Exercise,* 12: 153-158, 1980.

Hermansen. L. Anaerobic energy release. *Med. Sci. Sports,* 1: 32-38, 1969.

Heyters, C. and J.R. Poortmans. Evaluation de la capacité anaérobique: étude de la reproductibilité et de la validité d'un test de laboratoire. *Can. J. Appl. Sport Sci.,* 2: 183-187, 1977.

Hill, A.V., C.N.H. Long and H. Lupton. Muscular exercise, lactic acid and the supply and utilization of oxygen. Part IV-VI. *Proc. Roy. Soc. London, B.,* 96: 438-475, 1924.

Hollmann, W. *Höchst-und Dauerleistungsfähigkeit des Sportlers.* München, J.A. Barth, 1963.

Howald, H., G. von Glutz and R. Billeter. Energy stores and substrates utilization in muscle during exercise. In: *3rd International Symposium on Biochemistry of Exercise.* F. Landry and W.A.R. Orban (eds). Miami, Symposia Specialists, 1978, pp. 75-86.

Huckabee, W.E. Relationships of pyruvate and lactate during anaerobic metabolism. I. Effects of infusion of pyruvate or glucose and of hyperventilation. *J. Clin. Invest.,* 37: 244-254, 1958.

Inbar, O. and O. Bar-Or. The effects of intermittent warm-up on 7-9 year old boys. *Eur. J. Appl. Physiol.,* 34: 81-89, 1975.

Inbar, O. and O. Bar-Or. Relationships of anaerobic and aerobic arm and leg capacities to swimming performance of 8-12 year old children. In: *Limites de la capacité physique chez l'enfant.* H. Lavallée and R.J. Shephard (eds.) Québec, Editions du Pélican, 1977, pp. 157-159.

Jetté, M., J.S. Thoden and A. Reed. Les bases scientifiques de l'évaluation périodique. *Mouvement* (Spécial Hockey 2) 1975, pp. 99-104.

Jorfeldt, L., A. Juhlin-Dannfelt and J. Karlsson. Lactate release in relation to tissue lactate in human skeletal muscle during exercise. *J. Appl. Physiol.,* 44: 350-352, 1978.

Kalamen, J. *Measurement of maximum muscular power in man.* Doctoral dissertation, Ohio State University, 1968.

Karlsson, J. Muscle ATP, CP, and lactate in submaximal and maximal exercise. In: *Muscle metabolism during exercise. Advances in experimental medicine and biology.* B. Pernow and G. Saltin (eds). New York, Plenum Press, 1971, pp. 383-393.

Katch, V. Body weight, leg volume, leg weight and leg density as determiners of short duration work performance on the bicycle ergometer. *Med. Sci. Sports,* 6: 267-270, 1974.

Katch, V.L. and A. Weltman. Interrelationship between anaerobic power output, anaerobic capacity and aerobic power. *Ergonomics,* 22: 325-332, 1979.

Keul, J. The relationship between circulation and metabolism during exercise. *Med. Sci. Sports,* 5: 209-219, 1973.

Kindermann, W. and J. Keul. Lactate acidosis with different forms of sports activities. *Can. J. Appl. Sport Sci.,* 2: 177-182, 1977.

Klausen, K., K. Piehl and B. Saltin. Muscle glycogen stores and capacity for anaerobic work. In: *Metabolic adaptation to prolonged physical exercise.* H. Howald and J.R. Poortmans (eds). Basel, Birkhäuser, 1975, pp. 127-129.

Knowlton, R.G., K.J. Ackerman, P.I. Fitzgerald, S.W. Wilde and M.V. Tahamont. Physiological and performance characteristics of United States championship class orienteers. *Med. Sci. Sports Exercise,* 12: 164-169, 1980.

Knuttgen, H.G. Oxygen debt, lactate, pyruvate, and excess lactate after muscular work. *J. Appl. Physiol.,* 17: 639-644, 1962.

Larivière, G. and P. Godbout. *Mesure de la condition physique et de l'efficacité technique de joueurs de hockey sur glace. Normes pour différentes catégories de joueurs.* Québec, Editions du Pélican, 1976.

Margaria, R., P. Aghemo and E. Rovelli. Measurement of muscular power (anaerobic) in man. *J. Appl. Physiol.,* 21: 1662-1664, 1966.

Margaria, R., H.T. Edwards and D.B. Dill. The possible mechanism of contracting and paying the oxygen debt and the role of lactic acid in muscular contraction. *Am. J. Physiol.,* 106: 689-715, 1933.

Marrin, D.A., M.T. Sharratt and A.W. Taylor. A fitness profile for Canadian elite wrestlers. A mimeographed report, Canadian Amateur Wrestling Association, 1980.

Mayers, N. and B. Gutin. Physiological characteristics of elite prepubertal cross-country runners. *Med. Sci. Sports,* 11: 172-176, 1979.

Paterson, D.H., D.A. Cunningham and J.M. Bonk. Anaerobic capacity of athletic males aged 10, 15 and 21 years. Abstract of a paper presented at the International Symposium on Growth and Development of the Child, Trois-Rivières, 1980.

Poole, G.W., B.J. Crépin and M. Sévigny. Physiological characteristics of elite synchronized swimmers. *Can. J. Appl. Sport Sci.,* 5: 156-160, 1980.

Saltin, B. and J. Karlsson. Muscle glycogen utilization during work of different intensities. In: *Muscle metabolism during exercise. Advances in experimental medicine and biology.* B. Pernow and B. Saltin (eds). New York, Plenum Press, 1971, pp. 289-305.

Sawka, M.N., M.V. Tahamont, P.I. Fitzgerald, D.S. Miles and R.G. Knowlton. Alactic capacity and power, reliability and interpretation. *Eur. J. Appl. Physiol.,* 45: 109-116, 1980.

Simoneau, J.A., G. Lortie, M.R. Boulay and C. Bouchard. Tests of anaerobic alactacid and lactacid capacities: description and reliability (submitted for publication).

Song, T.M.K., A side-step test for a field test of anaerobic capacity. (In preparation). 1982.

Szögÿ, A. and G. Cherebetiu. Minutentest auf dem Fahrradergometer zur Bestimmung der anaerober Kapazität. *Eur. J. Appl. Physiol.,* 33: 171-176, 1974.

Tesch, P., B. Sjödin and J. Karlsson. Relationship between lactate accumulation, LDH activity, LDH isozyme and fiber type distribution in human skeletal muscle. *Acta Physiol. Scand.,* 103: 40-46, 1978.

Thomson, J.M. Prediction of anaerobic capacity: A performance test employing an optimal exercise stress. *Can. J. Appl. Sport Sci.,* 6(1): 16-20, 1981.

Thomson, J.M., G.M. Andrew and K.J. Garvie. A field test for determination of anaerobic capacity. A report to the Planning, Research and Evaluation Directorate, Fitness and Amateur Sport. Project No. 77-31, 1980.

CHAPTER SIX | Kinanthropometry

W.D. Ross • M.J. Marfell-Jones
with contributions by D.A. Bailey, J.E.L. Carter, J.P. Clarys, J.A.P. Day,
D.T. Drinkwater, R.M. Leahy, A.D. Martin, R.L. Mirwald, D.R. Stirling,
A.S. Vajda-Janyk, R. Ward

INTRODUCTION

Kinanthropometry: the quantitative link between structure and function. Kinanthropometry is an emerging scientific specialization having to do with the application of measurement to appraise human size, shape, proportion, composition, maturation, and gross function. It is a basic discipline for problem-solving in matters related to growth, exercise, performance, and nutrition.

KINANTHROPOMETRY

The quantitative interface between anatomy and performance

IDENTIFICATION	SPECIFICATION	APPLICATION	RELEVANCE
Kinanthropometry MOVEMENT HUMAN MEASUREMENT	For the study of human SIZE SHAPE PROPORTION COMPOSITION MATURATION GROSS FUNCTION	to help understand GROWTH EXERCISE PERFORMANCE NUTRITION	with implications for MEDICINE EDUCATION GOVERNMENT with respect for individual rights in the service of humankind.

The area has been defined as the quantitative interface between anatomy and physiology. It puts the individual athlete into objective focus and provides a clear appraisal of his or her structural status at any given time, or, more importantly, provides for quantification of differential growth and training influences (see Ross et al., 1982a).

MEASUREMENT OF STATUS AND CHANGE

Cross-Sectional Evaluation

If we wish to know how typical a youngster is for his or her age, we need to make a comparison with a representative sample which includes subjects with size and maturational variance characteristics of those in the particular sex and age range.

Fortunately, in Canada, with the expected resolution of the *Canada Fitness Survey*, we shall have superb normative data from 23,512 occupants, age 6 to 69 years old, from 13,440 households selected by geographical criteria from the whole country (Canada Fitness Survey, 1982).

Limited athletic norms are available from the world literature. Of particular interest are the height, weight, and ponderal index summaries by Hirata (1980), the anthropometric summaries from 1968 Mexico Olympic Games data by de Garay et al. (1974), and the 1976 Montreal Olympic Games data by Carter et al. (1982).

Included in this manual are updated specifications of measures and their standard deviations for a unisex reference human, or Phantom, originally described by Ross and Wilson (1974), reference data from a cross-sectional sampling of boys and girls age 6 to 18 years, and a tri-university sample of men and women for use as control data where similar data assemblies are unavailable (see section on *DATA MANAGEMENT — Resolution*).

Longitudinal Evaluation

Longitudinal Analysis

Longitudinal evaluations give an indication of *changing status* reflecting the endowment of the individual and growth and training influences.

Growth velocity curves can be constructed when one makes appropriate corrections for the time of the measurement occasions. Typical stature velocity curves for boys and girls are shown in Figures 6.1 and 6.2.

It should be recognized that these curves are maturity adjusted and represent centile values for stature. No child is typical in all parameters. Thus, it is necessary to construct individual growth curves which then can be compared to norms (see section on *MATURATION — Tri-dimensional Computer Graphics in Growth Curve Analysis*).

Frequency of Measurement

Stature measurements taken every three months, such as on the first weekday of September, December, March, and June, facilitate the derivation of velocity curves. However, stature data as infrequent as once a year are still of value. Occasionally, daily weight records may be useful in assessing compositional changes accompanying heavy training or dietary intervention. For monitoring growth, however, monthly or quarter-yearly weight records are satisfactory for most purposes.

Precision and Accuracy

In assessing individual status with respect to a particular norm, it is necessary that a high level of *precision* and *accuracy* be attained by the measurer. Precision is a matter of how consistent a measurer is with himself (intra-observer reliability) or with other measurers (inter-observer reliability). Accuracy is a matter of how closely obtained measures conform to *true* or *ideal* measures.

For example: if a measurer follows the Interna-

tional Biological Programme (IBP) recommended technique for shoulder, or biacromial breadth, the subject is measured with the shoulders rounded forward to give a maximal value (Weiner and Lourie, 1981). If a measurer uses the International Working Group on Kinanthropometry (IWGK) technique recommended in this manual, the subject is measured in an erect posture.

If the measurers had perfect precision in each technique, the IBP measure would always be greater than the IWGK measure. Thus, by IWGK standards, the IBP measure would be precise but inaccurate.

In longitudinal analyses, if one is primarily interested in growth rates or change in status, the major concern is that of precision. Provided one is absolutely precise in measurement, it is relatively unimportant which particular technique is employed to determine velocity values, since systematic differences tend to be consistent.

Investigators who wish to compare data to norms must have adequate *precision and accuracy* or have adequate precision and *know how their technique differs from that employed in the normative sample*. Thus, the matter of specification of landmarks and adherence to explicit technique as discussed in the sections on *SOMATYPE* and *MATURATION* is crucial in interpretation of data.

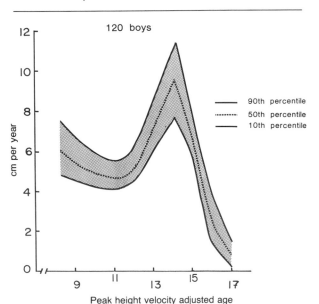

Fig. 6.1   Longitudinal stature velocity curves for boys. Saskatchewan Growth Study. Bailey and Mirwald.

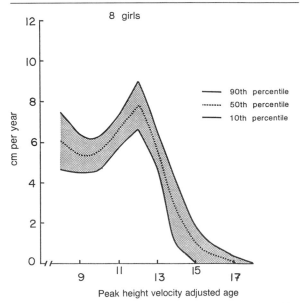

Fig. 6.2   Mixed-longitudinal stature velocity curves for girls. Saskatchewan Growth Study. Bailey and Mirwald.

ANTHROPOMETRY

Ostensibly, anthropometry is simple. In reality, it is not. Mastery of accurate measurement requires rigorous training and strict adherence to specified techniques.

Protocol

The measurement protocol outlined in this section is based on the deliberations of a Leon and Theta Koerner Foundation Study Group and specification of landmarks and conventions by Ross et al. (1978). The items have been selected because of the substantial data assemblies on Olympic athletes, particularly those in the 1968 Mexico Olympic Games reported by de Garay et al. (1974) and the 1976 Montreal Olympic Games (Borms et al., 1979; Carter et al., 1982). The items include all those taught in International Certification Courses in Kinanthropometry sponsored by the International Working Group on Kinanthropometry (endorsed by the Research Committee of the International Council in Sport and Physical Education, N.G.O., A-level committee, U.N.E.S.C.O.). In addition, items from the Canada Fitness Survey have been included to permit comparison of the above data to Canadian demographic norms.

The data from the recommended protocol provides for derivation of Heath-Carter somatotypes, Behnke somatograms, proportionality profiles and body composition estimates which can provide interpretive models.

Conventions and Landmarks

Because the body can assume a variety of postures, anthropometric description always is in reference to a *standard anatomical position*. This is where the subject is oriented to a standing position with head and eyes directed forward, upper limbs hanging by the sides with the palms forward, thumbs pointing away from the sides with fingers pointing directly downward, and the feet together with the toes pointing directly forward.

Three primary planes, as shown in Figure 6.3, describe position:

1. *Anteroposterior or sagittal plane.* This runs parallel to the vertical plane, which divides the body into right and left portions. The plane which divides the body into right and left halves is termed the *midsagittal plane*.

2. *Frontal or coronal plane.* This runs at right angles to the sagittal plane, dividing the body into front and rear portions.

3. *Transverse plane.* This runs at right angles to the other two planes, dividing the body into upper and lower portions.

Axes of the body are formed by the intersection of planes as follows:

a) Lateral axis is formed by an intersection of a frontal and a transverse plane.

b) Longitudinal axis is formed by an intersection of an anteroposterior and a frontal plane.

c) Anteroposterior or sagittal axis is formed by an intersection of a sagittal and a transverse plane.

The landmarks used are basically those defined by Ross et al. (1978), with additions as illustrated in Figure 6.4.

VERTEX (v). The most superior point on the skull, in the midsagittal plane, when the head is held in the Frankfort plane.

GNATHION (gn). Fr.: point mentonnier. Chin. The most inferior border of the mandible in the midsagittal plane.

SUPRASTERNALE (sst). Fr.: fourchette sternale. Suprasternal notch. The superior border of

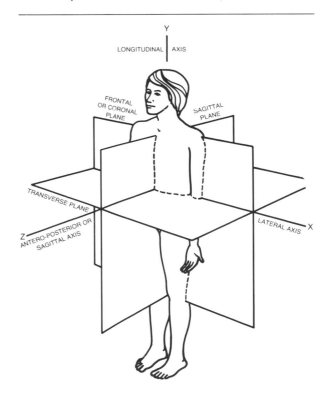

Fig. 6.3   Three primary planes.

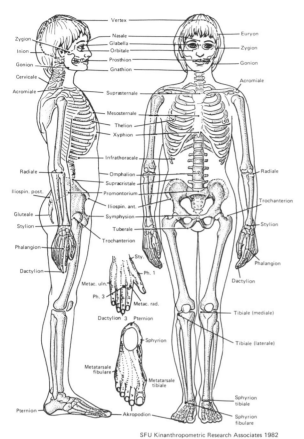

SFU Kinanthropometric Research Associates 1982

Fig. 6.4   Principal kinanthropometric landmarks.

the sternal notch (or incisura jugularis) in the midsagittal plane.

MESOSTERNALE (mst). Point located on the corpus sterni at the intersect of the midsagittal plane and the horizontal plane at the midlevel of the IV chondrosternal articulation.

EPIGASTRALE (eg). Point located on anterior surface of the trunk at the intersection of the midsagittal plane and the transverse plane through the most inferior point on the tenth ribs.

THELION (th). Breast nipple.

OMPHALION (om). Midpoint of navel or umbilicus.

SYMPHYSION (sy). Fr.: bord supérieur de la symphyse pubienne. The superior border of the symphysis pubis at the midsagittal plane. This is located by having the subject place his index fingers about four centimeters apart and proceed downward from the navel, palpating the abdominal wall gently until the bony surface of the pubis is

located. The anthropometrist can then palpate the "subject-located" landmark with his left thumb, avoiding the foreside of the subject's symphysis and genital parts which are inferior to the landmark. Generally, the landmark is at the upper level of the pubic hair zone and can be located through light clothing without difficulty.

ACROMIALE (a). Acromial point. The point at the superior and external border of the acromial process when the subject is standing erect with relaxed arms. This definition is in accord with the 1912 Geneva Convention (Stewart, 1952) but is not identical with "the most lateral" description of Martin and Saller (1957) or the "inferior-external border" found in the IBP Handbook (Weiner and Lourie, 1969). Location technique — see *Specification for Marking the Subject*, below.

RADIALE (r). The point at the upper and lateral border of the head of the radius. Location technique — see section *Specification for Marking the Subject*.

STYLION (sty). Fr.: apophyse styloide. The most distal point of the styloid process of the radius. It is located in the so-called "anatomical snuff box" (Fr.: tabatière anatomique), the triangular area formed when the thumb is extended and defined by the raised tendons of abductor pollicus longus and extensor pollicus brevis laterally and extensor pollicus longus medially. For measurements on the ulna, the stylion ulnare can be used.

DACTYLION (da). Fr.: extrémité intérieur du doigt medius. Tip of the middle finger. The most distal point of the middle finger or digit when the arm is hanging and the fingers are stretched downwards. The corresponding tips of the other fingers are designated dactylion I, II, IV, and V.

METACARPALE RADIALE (mr). The most medial point of the distal head of the fifth metacarpal of the outstretched hand, i.e. on the ulnar side of the hand.

ILIOCRISTALE (ic). Fr.: crête iliaque. The most lateral point of the crista iliaca. This landmark is encompassed when obtaining biiliocristal breadth with an anthropometer.

ILIOSPINALE (is). Fr.: épine iliaque antéro-supérieure. The anterior superior iliac spine. The designated landmark is the undersurface of the tip of the anterior superior spine and not the most frontally curved aspect.

TROCHANTERION (tro). The most superior point on the greater trochanter of the femur, not the most lateral point.

TIBIALE MEDIALE (tm). Tibiale internum. Fr.:

ligne articulaire du genou. Superior extremity of the tibia. The most proximal point of the margo glenoidalis on the medial border of the head of the tibia. To find the tibiale, the upper border of the tibia is located by palpating the quadriceps tendon at the distal end of the patella. This may be facilitated by having the subject slightly flex his leg. The index finger is moved inward pressing the skin to locate the tibial point of the articulation at the frontal border of the ligamentum collaterale tibiale. The level at this point should be marked as the reference.

TIBIALE LATERALE (tl). This point corresponds to the tibiale mediale above but is located on the lateral border of the head of the tibia. It is above, and not to be confused with, the more inferior capitulum fibulare. Location technique — see section *Specification for Marking the Subject*.

Both tibiale mediale and tibiale laterale are situated in practically the same transverse plane.

SPHYRION (sph). Malleolare mediale or malleolare internum. The most distal tip of the malleolare medialis (tibialis). This landmark may be located most easily from beneath and dorsally. It is the distal tip and not the outermost point of the malleolus.

SPHYRION FIBULARE (sph f). Malleolare laterale or malleolare externum. The most distal tip of the malleolare laterale (fibularis). The sphyrion fibulare is more distal than the sphyrion tibiale.

PTERNION (pte). The most posterior point on the heel of the foot when the subject is standing.

AKROPODION (ap). The most anterior point on the toe of the foot when the subject is standing. This may be the first or second phalanx. The subject's toenail may have to be clipped to make a measurement.

METATARSALE TIBIALE (mt t). The most medial point on the head of metatarsal I of the foot when the subject is standing.

METATARSALE FIBULARE (mt f). The most lateral point of the head of metatarsal V when the subject is standing.

CERVICALE (c). The most posterior point on the spinous process of the seventh cervical vertebra. To locate this landmark, the subject nods his head forward; the spinous process of the seventh cervical vertebra moves away from the spinous process of the usually more prominent first thoracic vertebra; once the cervicale is located, the subject assumes an erect standing position and its location is marked.

GLUTEALE (ga). Midgluteal arch. This point is at the sacrococcygeal fusion in the midsagittal plane. It is located by placing the thumb at the top of the gluteal furrow and palpating in a downward direction with the thumb. The fingers should be spread upwards over the lumbar region of the subject and the landmark can be located with minimal adjustment of clothing.

Instruments

In terms of scientific and medical equipment anthropometric instruments are reasonably inexpensive and durable.

The complete anthropometric kit recommended for use in this manual is shown in Figure 6.5. The items include:

1. Lufkin retractable metric measuring tape (Y22M) with adapted footpiece used to measure stature.

2. Broca plane: a simple triangular head board.

3. Anthropometric tape. The tape of choice is Keuffel and Esser Whyteface steel tape (No. 860358). A blackface Lufkin tape (146 ME) is a reasonable substitute. Other tapes may be used; they should, however, have all of the following characteristics:

a) Non-extensibility (steel): if other materials are used, the tape must be frequently examined to ensure accurate readings.

b) Flexibility: ideally no wider than 7 mm.

c) Ease of reading: calibrated in metric units with unequivocal identification of the centimeter mark (tapes with English and metric scales on the same side of the tape are inadequate).

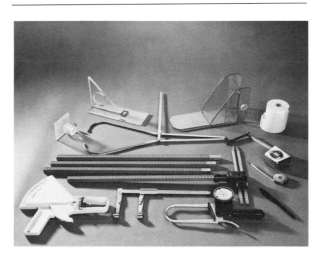

Fig. 6.5 Complete anthropometric kit.

d) A stub: before the zero line to facilitate manipulation.

e) Freedom from spring or other devices ostensibly aimed at achieving a constant pressure (see section *General Instructions for Obtaining Girths*).

f) Absolute accuracy of scale. (This must be checked. In evaluating tapes for the Canada Fitness Survey two supposedly reputable brands were incorrectly calibrated and one appeared to be stretchable.)

4. Anthropometer. The instrument of choice is the Siber-Hegner GPM anthropometer of the Martin type used with a footplate as illustrated. The kit should include two straight branches. If it is to be used in lieu of a wide-spreading caliper for anterior-posterior chest depth, it also should have two recurved branches with olive tips. The Harpenden anthropometer which features a digital counter may be used. It, however, requires adding constants for projected heights and some servicing of mechanical parts.

5. Skinfold calipers. The instrument of choice is the Harpenden caliper (British Indicators Ltd., Acrewood Way, Hatfield Road, St. Albans, Herts, England) which is virtually standard in Canada. Alternate models are the Lange caliper (Cambridge Scientific Industries, Cambridge, Maryland) and the inexpensive plastic Slimguide caliper (Creative Health Products, 5148 Saddle Ridge Road, Plymouth, Michigan 48170). The Lange caliper yields approximately similar values compared to the Harpenden caliper whereas the Slimguide yields systematically smaller values. All three in the hands of a trained anthropometrist are highly reliable. For the eight sites recommended in this manual, the following regression equation may be used to translate Slimguide (S) values to comparable Harpenden (H) values (median values of triple measures, n = 29, r = 0.993, S.E. = 0.68). This equation applies to Slimguide caliper models which do not have a zero stop.

$$H = 1.03 (S) + 0.64$$

6. Bone calipers. Adapted Mitutoyo bone calipers as described by Carter (1980) are recommended for humerus and femur widths. These calipers have extended branches with round pressure plates 15 mm in diameter. The inside diameter branches are removed and the locking device is fixed to permit easy manipulation.

7. Widespreading calipers. The large widespreading calipers (Siber-Hegner, GPM) are the instrument of choice for A-P chest depth. However, anthropometers with recurved branches may be used as a substitute.

8. Weighing machine. The instrument of choice is a portable beam-type balance, calibrated in kilograms and tenths of kilograms. (Homs full capacity beam scale — general weighing scale, 150 kg) This model was used in the Canada Fitness Survey. A substitute spring type balance (SECA), however, has been used in field studies. The onus is on the investigator to make sure the weighing machines are calibrated and do not vary in the course of the measurement program.

9. In laboratory operations a wall-mounted parallax-correcting stadiometer, described by Ross (1976), or ball-bearing digital wall-mounted, portable stadiometer, or sitting stadiometer (Harpenden) may be substituted for the Lufkin tape specified above.

10. Anthropometric box. A 50 × 40 × 30 cm box may be used for posing the subject to obtain leg measurements E 32 to 35, and items in G (Figure 6).

11. Measuring platform. In many field test situations floors are not level or are uncomfortable to the barefoot subject. A useful optional piece of equipment is a one meter square wooden 5-ply platform which may be leveled by wooden shims.

12. Other alternate equipment includes: screwdrivers, pliers and allen key to service anthropometric equipment; a carpenter's spirit-level; standard weights for calibration of balance-beam weigh machine which serves, in turn, to calibrate the spring scale, and a hand calculator such as a Texas Instrument 55 which provides a capacity for immediate hand calculation of data.

A simple field test calibration for skinfold calipers is to fix the instrument in a vise and suspend weights from the lower jaw. The caliper should be adjusted so that the jaws remain open in any position when the calibration weight shown in Figure 6.6 is used.

Proforma

The proforma shown as Figure 6.7 facilitates systematic data collection by a single anthropometrist and various deployments, including a seven-station multiple line procedure.

In routine operation, the form is reproduced providing for a non-carbon first, yellow second, and pink third copy page. The first page goes to the computer operator for inputting and then to the

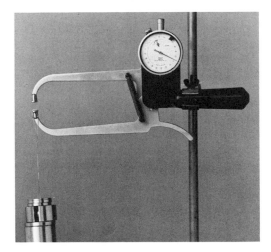

Fig. 6.6 Skinfold caliper calibration.

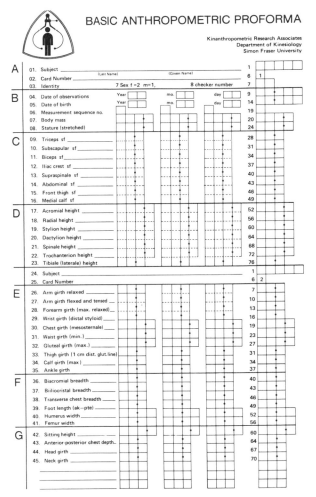

Fig. 6.7 Basic kinanthropometric proforma.

permanent file for the primary investigator. The second page is routinely filed in the laboratory and thus is a physically-separated, replicated file in case of loss or misplacement of the first copy. The third copy usually is given to the coach, subject, or parents and thus is available for verification by anyone who cares to replicate measures.

Section A of the proforma provides for subject identification. This section and items 04 and 05 of section B may be filled out in advance of the measurement occasion. The date of birth and measurement occasion are expressed as year, month, and day and then converted to decimals by referring to Appendix 6.1.

For items 07 and 08 in section B and all other sections, four columns are provided. In routine operation where individual interpretations rather than group analyses are involved, the whole sequence is completed, and then replicated twice. This provides three sets of data for each item and helps in error control as discussed in the section *Data Collection and Error Control*. The fourth column provides for entry of median values or, if only one series is made, the data can be entered in this column.

Techniques

Anthropometry appears deceptively simple. Mastery, however, is somewhat analogous to playing a musical instrument with style and grace. With some formal training and persistent practice, it can be easy and enjoyable and can produce amazingly accurate data. The development of an anthropometrist's touch seldom is achieved without extensive practice. It varies from individual to individual, but most seem to achieve reasonable competence after triple-measurement and spot-checking for systematic error with criterion anthropometry measures on 100 or so subjects.

A "criterion anthropometrist" by definition is one who purportedly does not make systematic errors from a prescribed technique. As a service to the international scientific community, the International Working Group in Kinanthropometry holds certification courses and workshops. These are designed primarily for established investigators to learn IWGK protocols and assess systematic differences with local and other protocols.

In the measurement sequence, only *right* side values of the subject are taken in surveys. The convention of the IBP is to use *left* side; however, since kinanthropometrists and sportspeople are primarily interested in the most-dominant side, the right is preferred. When there is a question of bilateral asymmetry, however, *both* sides should be taken. In some athletes, asymmetry is an important factor in their structural appraisal. This may be of major concern in appraisal of trauma in tennis players, runners, and skaters.

Specification for Marking the Subject

a) ACROMIALE (a): the point at the superior and external border of the scapula.

The procedure is to locate first the most superior border, and then the most lateral aspect. The subject stands erect, arms relaxed. The marker stands behind the subject and locates the acromion by palpating laterally along the spinous process of the scapula. A marking pencil as a straight edge is applied to the lateral aspect of the acromion process to depress tissue and identify the superior border. The most lateral point on the superior border is identified, the pencil pressure is removed, the landmark is confirmed on the uncompressed surface and marked, then re-identified as a check.

b) RADIALE (r): the point at the upper and lateral border of the head of the radius.

Using his left thumb or index finger, the anthropometrist palpates downward in the lower portion of the lateral dimple of the elbow. Slight pronation/supination of the forearm is reflected by a rotary movement of the head of the radius. Marking and checking the landmark are done as above.

c) MID-ACROMIALE-RADIALE ARM AND TRICEPS SITES:

A line is marked horizontal to the long axis of the humerus at the mid-acromiale-radiale distance, as determined by an anthropometric tape. The horizontal line is extended to the posterior surface of the arm, where a vertical line at the most posterior surface is made to intersect with the horizontal line, to mark the site where the triceps skinfold is raised. The biceps site is marked anteriorly.

d) STYLION (sty): the most distal point of the processus styloidus radius.

This is located in the so-called "anatomical snuff box" identified by extending the thumb. The anthropometrist places the nail of his left thumb or index finger in the triangular space outlined by the

muscle tendons. The landmark is palpated by having the subject relax while the anthropometrist slightly manipulates his hand from side to side. Marking and checking the landmark are done as above.

e) MESOSTERNALE (mst): the point on the corpus sterni at the intersection of the midsagittal and horizontal planes, at the midlevel of the fourth chondrosternal articulation.

A two-handed palpation method provides for rapid location of the landmark. The anthropometrist places his index fingers on the top of the clavicles while the thumbs locate the first costal spaces, thus encompassing the first ribs. He then moves his index fingers to replace the thumbs which are lowered to the second intercostal spaces to identify the second ribs. The procedure is repeated for the third and fourth ribs. The landmark is at the mid-point of the sternum at the level of the center of the articulation of the 4th rib with the sternum.

f) SPINALE (spi): the inferior aspect of the tip of the anterior superior iliac spine.

The subject stands on his left foot, lifts his right heel and rotates the femur outward. The anthropometrist grasps the hip with his left hand, and locates the landmark with his thumb. Since the sartorius muscle arises from the spinale, slight movement of the thigh enables identification of the muscle, which can then be followed to the landmark. Once the landmark is identified, the subject stands erect, with feet together, while the spinale is marked and checked.

g) TROCHANTERION (tro): the most superior point on the greater trochanter of the femur.

The subject takes a short forward stride and rests his foot on a raised object about 15 cm high. The anthropometrist stands behind the subject, stabilizing him with his left hand, and starts palpating with his right hand on the lateral aspect of the gluteal muscle, on a line with the long axis of the femur. Once the greater trochanter is identified by firm downward pressure, the subject carefully assumes the erect stance with weight equally distributed on each foot, and the toes pointing directly forward. The anthropometrist then palpates upward to locate the most superior point on the greater trochanter. As usual, the pressure is released and reapplied so that the mark can be made on an undisturbed skin surface.

h) TIBIALE LATERALE (externum) (tl): the most proximal point of the margo glenoidalis of the lateral border of the head of the tibia.

It is often easier to locate the landmark by having the subject flex his leg at the knee, or sit down. The tibiale laterale can be located as follows: (1) find the depression or dimple in the knee, bounded by a triad of prominences — epicondylar femur, antero/lateral portion of the head of the tibia, and the head of the fibula; (2) from this orientation, the anthropometrist presses inward, locating the border of the tibia; (3) the anthropometrist then palpates posteriorly along the border until he locates the landmark, which is the most superior point. This point is at least one-third of the distance from the anterior to the posterior surface of the knee joint. Once the landmark is identified, the subject stands erect and the mark is made when the border is felt by the finger or thumb nail.

The tibiale laterale is approximately in the same transverse plane as the tibiale mediale.

Specification for Obtaining Body Mass and Stretch Stature

Body Mass: Ideally, body weight should be obtained on an accurately calibrated beam-type balance and recorded to the nearest 0.1 kg. The subject should be weighed nude or in clothing of known weight so a correction to nude weight can be made. The most stable values for monitoring weight change are those obtained routinely in the morning, twelve hours after having ingested food, and after voiding. However, such exact control is not generally necessary for growth records. For most purposes, a calibrated spring scale with measurement made to the nearest 0.5 kg is satisfactory.

Stature (stretch): There are four general techniques for measuring stature which yield slightly different values. These are: freestanding stature, stature against the wall, recumbent length and stretch stature.

The standard method for this manual is stretch stature. An explicit description of the selected technique and strict adherence to it are important.

The measurement is normally made with the device known as a stadiometer, although a constructed device is not essential. The instrument can be fairly elaborate, feature ball-bearing counter-weighted headboards and digital readouts, or it can be little more than two wooden planes at right angles. The practice of using a wooden rectangular chalk box and pencil marks on the door jamb can yield satisfactory results. A carpenter's re-

tractable measuring tape with footpiece can be used to measure the length from the floor to mark. Unfortunately, the typical doctor's office stadiometer attached to a beam-type scale is inadequate and must NOT be used for classification purposes.

The technique requires precise positioning of the subject in order to obtain useful measurements. The measurement is taken as the maximum distance from the floor to the vertex of the head. Technically, the vertex is defined as the highest point on the skull when the head is held in the Frankfort Plane. This position is achieved as indicated in Figure 6.8, when the line joining the orbitale to the tragion is horizontal or at right angles to the long axis of the body. The orbitale is located on the lower or most inferior position on the margin of the eye socket. The tragion is the notch above or superior to the flap of the ear, at the superior aspect of the zygomatic bone. This position corresponds almost exactly to the visual axis when the subject is looking directly ahead.

In making the stature measurement, the measurer has the barefoot subject stand erect with heels together and arms hanging naturally by the sides. The heels, buttocks, upper part of the back and usually, but not necessarily, the back of the head are in contact with the vertical wall. The subject is instructed to "look straight ahead" and "take a deep breath." One of the measurers ensures that the subject's heels are not elevated while the other measurer applies stretch force, by cupping the subject's head and applying gentle traction at the mastoid processes. The first measurer then brings the headpiece firmly down in contact with the vertex and makes a pencil mark on the paper tape level with the underside of the headpiece. The subject then steps away from the wall, the headpiece is removed and the vertical distance from floor to pencil mark is measured with the retractable metal tape stadiometer (see section on *Instruments*). The measurement is read to the nearest 0.1 cm.

General Instructions for Obtaining Skinfold Thicknesses

Instrument: Harpenden skinfold caliper (or substitutes, see section on *Instruments*). The instrument is designed to provide a constant pressure of 10.0 g·mm^{-2} of the caliper face at all thicknesses. The dial is calibrated in 0.2 mm increments. It may be read, by interpolation, to the nearest 0.1 mm.

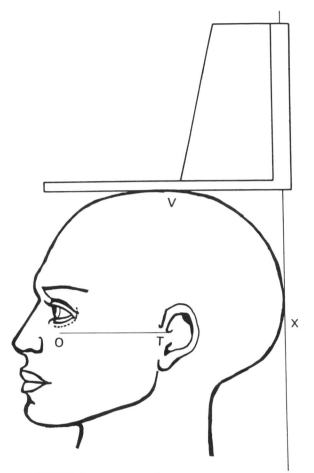

ORBITALE: Lower margin of eye socket

TRAGION: Notch above tragus of ear or at upper margin of zygomatic bone at that point

FRANKFORT PLANE: Orbitale-tragion line horizontal

VERTEX: Highest point on skull when head is held in Frankfort plane.

Fig. 6.8   Frankfort Plane.

Technique: The caliper is used to obtain a skinfold thickness. This includes a double layer of skin and the underlying adipose tissue, but not the muscle. The skinfold is raised by the pinching, slightly rolling action of the left thumb and index finger. The grasp is large enough to get a complete double layer. The fold is grasped firmly and held throughout the measurement. The skinfold is raised at the designated site and the caliper is applied so that the near edge of the pressure plate is one centimeter from the lateral side of the controlling thumb and index finger. Care must be

taken to assure the caliper is applied at right angles to the fold at all times. The reading on the dial is taken after permitting full spring pressure of the instrument by a complete release of the caliper trigger. The investigator must allow time for the full pressure of the caliper to take effect, but not so long that the adipose tissue becomes "squeezed out" of the skinfold. Considerable practice is required to make this judgment for skinfolds of varying sizes and varying degrees of compressibility. The reading is made approximately two seconds after application, when the needle slows. In measuring obese subjects, firm pressure of the thumb and index finger helps reduce excessive movement of the indicator. When skinfold thicknesses are difficult to raise, the caliper can be forced to the muscle level and then slightly withdrawn when the fold is controlled by the grasp.

Sites (see Figure 6.9). All of the following measures are made on the *right* side of the body with the exception of the abdominal fold, which is made on the left side. The numbers refer to the Proforma (Figure 6.7).

09. *Triceps:* the caliper distance when applied one centimeter from the left thumb and index finger raising a vertical fold at the marked mid-acromiale-radiale line on the posterior surface of the arm.

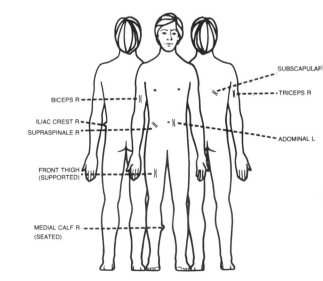

Fig. 6.9   Skinfold sites.

10. *Subscapular:* the caliper distance when applied one centimeter distally from the left thumb and index finger raising a fold beneath the inferior angle of the scapula in a direction running obliquely downwards at an angle of about 45 degrees from the horizontal.

11. *Biceps:* the caliper distance when applied one centimeter distally from the left thumb and index finger raising a vertical fold at the marked mid-acromiale-radiale line on the anterior surface of the right arm.

12. *Iliac crest:* the caliper distance when applied one centimeter anteriorly from the left thumb and index finger raising a fold immediately superior to the iliac crest at the mid-axillary line. The fold runs anteriorly downwards and usually is progressively smaller as one moves in this direction from the designated site.

13. *Supraspinale* (formerly Heath-Carter supraILiac): the caliper distance when applied one centimeter anteriorly from the left thumb and index finger raising a fold about seven centimeters above the spinale on a line to the anterior axillary border (armpit). The fold follows the natural fold lines running medially downwards at about a 45-degree angle from horizontal.

14. *Abdominal:* the caliper distance when applied one centimeter inferior to the left thumb and index finger raising a vertical fold which is raised 5 cm lateral to, and at the level of, the omphalion (midpoint of the navel).

15. *Front thigh:* the caliper distance when applied one centimeter distally to the left thumb and index finger raising a fold on the anterior of the right thigh along the long axis of the femur when the leg is flexed at an angle of 90 degrees at the knee by placing the foot on a box. The mid-thigh position for this measure is the estimated half-distance between the inguinal crease and anterior patella. In some subjects when the fold is difficult to raise, the grasp must be firm, calipers can be pushed to the muscle level and slightly retracted and the subject, himself, can assist by supporting the underside of the leg. In particularly heavy-thighed subjects, the anthropometrist can give further support to the underside of the leg by using his own knee and thigh. A further tactic is to have an assistant use two hands to raise the fold. The anthropometrist applies the caliper from the subject's right side when the assistant on his left raises the fold with his right thumb and index finger at the prescribed site; the anthropometrist positions the caliper and a second grasp of the fold is attempted with the assistant's right thumb and index finger one centimeter distal to the caliper. The measurement is made on the double grasped fold.

16. *Medial calf:* the caliper distance when applied one centimeter distal to the left thumb and index finger raising a vertical fold on the medial right calf at the estimated greatest circumference. This is easiest to obtain when the subject's leg is flexed to an angle of 90 degrees at the knee by placing the foot on a box.

General Instructions for Projected Lengths

Instrument: Siber-Hegner anthropometer with footplate.

Technique: The anthropometer is maneuvered so the extended branch, with a point at lower edge, is placed on the marked site. The level of the cursor can be adjusted by the anthropometrist's right hand, leaving his left hand free to check the landmark and stabilize the moveable branch. The anthropometrist holds the vertical shaft with his palm and fingers. His thumb extends upwards and manipulates the cursor to make the fine adjustment for the point of the branch.

During projected measures on the upper extremity, the subject should stand erect with the arms at the sides, palms against the thighs and fingers extended vertically downwards. It is essential in measuring upper extremity lengths that the shoulders of the subject maintain a constant position throughout the sequence. The anthropometer must be kept vertical for all projected measures. The point of the branch must be maneuvered to the exact site, and the level stabilized *before* the reading is made.

Lengths (see Figure 6.10). The numbers refer to the Proforma (Figure 6.7).

17. *Acromial height:* (ah) acromiale to base.

18. *Radial height:* (rh) radiale to base.

19. *Stylion height:* (sty h) stylion to base.

20. *Dactylion height:* (da h) dactylion to base. Special care must be taken to keep the hand straight and to avoid it following the curve of the thigh. As in all projected heights, the level of the landmark is at the point or lower edge of the anthropometer branch.

21. *Spinale height:* (spi h) spinale to base.

22. *Trochanterion height:* (tro h) trochanterion to base.

23. *Tibial (lateral) height:* (ti l) tibiale to base.

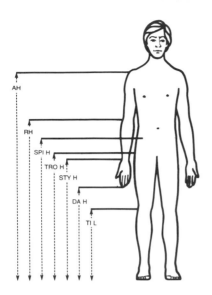

Fig. 6.10   Projected lengths (Landmarks, p. 78-79).

General Instructions for Obtaining Girths

Instrument: Flexible steel tape, calibrated in centimeters with millimeter gradations; 1.5 to 2.0 meters long with an end tab before the zero marking; enclosed in a case with a button spring release for retraction.

Technique: The metal case is held in the right hand throughout all the girth measurements. The girths are measured with the tape at right angles to the long axis of a bone or body segment. The tape is passed around the part and held so the stub end and the scale calibrations are in juxtaposition, i.e., one reads to a scale mark and not across a tape space. The reading edge of the tape is manipulated to the designated level, e.g., the marked mid-arm site. When measuring, the tape is pulled out of its housing and around the part by the left hand, which then transfers the stub end to the right hand. The tape is then controlled by the right hand which can pull it slightly to maintain it at the designated level. The left hand then resumes control of the stub end and can make any further adjustments to the tape. The so-called "cross-handed" technique is simply a matter of reaching across with the left hand and gripping the stub end of the tape with the thumb and index finger while the right hand similarly grasps the tape at the housing end. The tape is then brought into juxtaposition using the third

digit of each hand to control or make adjustments. The aim is to obtain the perimeter distance of the part with the tape in contact with, but not depressing, the fleshy contour. The development of this light touch requires considerable practice since the pressure on the tape is not constant, but is governed by the compressibility of the fleshy contour which varies among individuals.

Careful attention must be given to the girth specifications. The arm girth relaxed is at a designated and marked level whereas the flexed-and-tensed arm girth is obtained at the site of the greatest perimeter over volitionally-contracted musculature.

Technically good anthropometrists have economy of movement and precise control of the tape. This is only achieved by persistent practice under the tutelage of a criterion anthropometrist or by viewing video-tape records of the whole sequence and eliminating extraneous aspects.

Girths (Figure 6.11).

26. *Arm girth relaxed:* the perimeter distance of the right arm parallel to the long axis of the humerus when the subject is standing erect and the relaxed arm is hanging by the sides. The level of the tape is at the measured and marked mid-acromiale-radiale distance.

27. *Arm girth flexed and tensed:* the maximum circumference of the right arm raised to the horizontal position. The subject is encouraged to

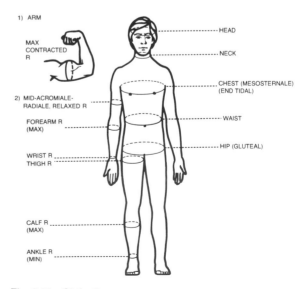

Fig. 6.11   Girth sites.

"make a muscle" by tensing and fully flexing his forearm at the elbow. In making this measurement, a preliminary flexing permits the investigator to adjust the tape to the maximal girth which is then achieved at a second trial where the subject is encouraged verbally "Up, up, up, up." This measure is obtained when the anthropometrist stands laterally to the right of the subject.

28. *Forearm girth:* the maximal girth of the right forearm when the hand is held palm up and relaxed. The measure is made no more distally than 6 cm from the radiale. In subjects with pronounced forearm development where the belly of the muscles is more distal than normal, a "true" maximal value will differ from the conventional forearm girth which is taken at the more proximal level.

29. *Wrist girth:* the perimeter of the right wrist taken distal to the styloid processes.

30. *Chest girth:* the subject slightly abducts his arms to permit the anthropometrist standing to his right facing him to pass the tape around his chest; the tape and housing is held in the right hand while the anthropometrist's left hand adjusts the tape at the subject's back to the horizontal level of the marked mesosternale. The cross-handed technique is used to put the tape scale in juxtaposition with the zero on the stub end of the tape. The reading is obtained at the end of a normal expiration (end tidal).

31. *Waist girth:* the perimeter at the level of the noticeable waist narrowing located approximately half way between the costal border and the iliac crest. In subjects where the waist is not apparent, an arbitrary waist measurement is made at this level.

32. *Gluteal girth (hip girth):* the perimeter at the level of the greatest posterior protuberance and at approximately the symphysion pubis level anteriorly. The subject during this measure stands erect, feet together, without volitionally contracting the gluteal muscles.

33. *Thigh girth:* the perimeter of the right thigh which is measured when the subject stands erect, legs slightly parted, weight equally distributed on both feet. The tape is raised to a level one to two centimeters below the gluteal line or the arbitrary join of the gluteal muscle protuberance with the thigh. A cross-handed technique is used to raise the tape to this level on the inner thigh then the tape is read when the stub end is brought in juxtaposition to the housing end. In this, the third digits are used to manipulate and fix the tape to assure the measure is made perpendicular to the long

axis of the femur.

34. *Calf girth:* with the subject in the same position as above, the tape is maneuvered to obtain the maximum perimeter of the calf. This measure is obtained by manipulation of the tape taking a series of girth measurements to assure the largest value. This is achieved by a relaxing and tightening of the tape with manipulation to various levels facilitated by the anthropometrist's third digits.

35. *Ankle girth:* the perimeter of the narrowest part of the lower leg superior to the sphyrion tibiale. From the side, because of the ovoid shape of the leg, this is slightly below the visual impression of the narrowest point. The tape is manipulated by loosening and tightening to obtain the minimal girth measure. In the process, the anthropometrist's third digits are used to maintain the perpendicular orientation of the tape to the long axis of the tibia.

General Instructions for Obtaining Breadths

Instrument: Siber-Hegner anthropometer used as a large sliding caliper; and small Mitutoyo adapted bone calipers.

Technique: the anthropometer must be assembled properly. The sliding branch should be on the right hand side of the anthropometrist. When closed the anthropometer indicator should read 0.7 mm (the small distance the branches are apart when fully closed).

Both the sliding and the bone calipers are held in the same manner. The branches are gripped by the thumb and the index finger and rest on the backs of the hands. The middle finger is used to locate the landmark. Firm pressure is applied to the branches.

The vernier scale on the smaller bone calipers can be read to the nearest 0.01 cm on some models and to the nearest 0.1 mm on others. Thus a typical value for the humerus might be 7.21 cm or 72.1 mm.

Breadths (Figure 6.12).

36. *Biacromial breadth:* the distance between the most lateral points on the acromion processes when the subject stands erect with the arms hanging loosely at the sides. The anthropometrist stands behind the subject, locates the sites with his third digit and applies the branches of the anthropometer used as a sliding caliper to the sites. The branches of the caliper point *upwards* at an angle of about 45 degrees from the horizontal to encompass the largest diameter between the

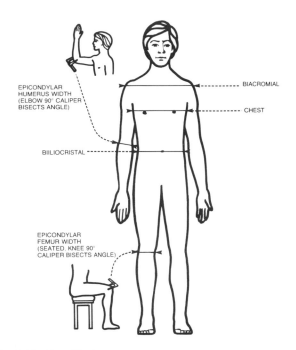

EPICONDYLAR
HUMERUS WIDTH
(ELBOW 90° CALIPER
BISECTS ANGLE)

BIACROMIAL

CHEST

BIILIOCRISTAL

EPICONDYLAR
FEMUR WIDTH
(SEATED. KNEE 90°
CALIPER BISECTS ANGLE)

Fig. 6.12   Breadth sites.

acromial processes. Firm pressure is applied to the branches over the acromial sites by the anthropometrist's index fingers.

37. *Biiliocristal breadth:* the distance between the most lateral points on the superior border of the iliac crest. The anthropometrist stands in front of the subject, locates the sites with his third digits and applies the branches of the anthropometer used as a sliding caliper to the sites. The branches of the caliper point *upwards* at an angle of about 45 degrees from the horizontal to encompass the largest diameter between the lateral aspects of the iliac crests. Firm pressure is applied to the branches over the iliac sites by the anthropometrist's index fingers.

38. *Transverse chest width:* the distance of the lateral aspect of the thorax at the level of the most lateral aspect of the fourth rib. This is obtained by applying the anthropometer used as a sliding caliper to the subject who is seated erect and faced by the anthropometrist. The caliper is applied at an angle of about 30 degrees *downward* from the horizontal avoiding both the pectoral and latissimus dorsi muscle contours. When the site is approximated, the anthropometrist removes his thumbs from the pinch grasp of the branches and

applies firm pressure with his index fingers. The measurement is made at the end of the normal expiratory excursion (end tidal).

39. *Footlength:* the distance between the akropodion and pternion obtained by the anthropometer used as a sliding caliper on the standing subject. The caliper is held parallel to the long axis of the foot. The anthropometrist holds the branch end of the caliper in his left hand, grasps the shaft with his right hand digits 2, 3, 4; in opposition to digit 5; while manipulating the cursor with his thumb. The sites are encompassed with minimal pressure.

40. *Biepicondylar humerus width:* the distance between medial and lateral epicondyles of the humerus when the arm is raised forward to the horizontal and the forearm is flexed to a right angle at the elbow. The small bone caliper is applied pointing *upwards* to bisect the right angle formed at the elbow. The epicondyles are palpated by the third digits starting proximal to the sites. The measured distance is somewhat oblique since the medial epicondyle is lower than the lateral. However, with the altered plane, the anthropometrist keeps the calipers as close to horizontal as possible while ensuring the pressure plates are applied firmly to the encompassed sites.

41. *Biepicondylar femur width:* the distance between medial and lateral epicondyles of the femur when the subject is seated and the leg is flexed at the knee to form a right angle with the thigh. The small bone caliper is applied pointing *downwards* to bisect the right angle formed at the knee. The epicondyles are palpated by the third digits starting proximal to the sites. The caliper pressure plates are applied firmly. If difficulty is encountered in locating the epicondyles, the third digits can search in a slightly circular motion and caliper pressure plates can be manipulated slightly to ensure the sites are encompassed.

General Instructions for Obtaining Sitting Height, A-P Chest Depth, Head Girth and Neck Girth (Figure 6.13)

42. *Sitting height:* the distance from the vertex to the base sitting surface when the seated subject is instructed to sit tall and gentle traction is applied to the mandible. This measurement is usually made when the subject is seated on a table with feet off the floor. When it is made on a box with the feet on the floor, care must be taken to ensure the subject does not push with the legs. AN ASSIST-

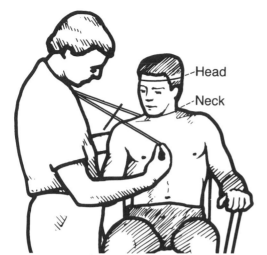

Fig. 6.13   Sites for A-P chest, head and neck measurements.

44. *Head girth:* maximum perimeter of the head when the tape is located immediately superior to the glabella point (mid-point between brow ridges). The tape is located perpendicular to the long axis of the seated subject whose head is oriented in the Frankfort Plane. Because of intervening hair, the usual light touch for girths is replaced by a firmer measure which crushes hair to minimize its influence.

45. *Neck girth:* the perimeter of the neck taken immediately superior to the larynx (Adam's apple). The tape is located perpendicular to the long axis of the neck of the seated subject when his head is oriented in the Frankfort Plane. The usual light anthropometric touch is applied to the tape.

DATA MANAGEMENT

Data Collection and Error Control

The sample data proforma provides three columns for three measurement series. Statistically, with replicated measures the mean serves as the most representative value. However, in anthropometry the hazards are two-fold: (1) blunders: misreading, voice error, auditory problem or recording mistake and (2) mislocated landmarks. These errors are occasionally gross. Hence, the selection of the median value is less influenced by these factors. Also, using the median value avoids arithmetic and round-off errors.

In operation, the anthropometrist and recorder act as a team, one measuring and clearly calling out the values: e.g., 169.2

"one, six, nine, point, two"

The other records the values and re-calls the digits as he writes them in the space provided.

Thus, all the measurer and recorder are required to know are zero and nine digits and this permits international teams to use any convenient language for simple counts.

The digits must be clearly formed. One is a straight line " I " not the European one " *1* " which can be confused with a seven or four. Similarly Western investigators should adopt the European "7" and not the 7 which is variously interpreted as a nine, four or one. Care must also be given to making zeros as "0" and not "*6*" or "*0*" which could be misinterpreted as a six or nine. In some items, the first space of the entry may be a zero, e.g., item 30, chest girth, should be 096.3. Thus, in a completed form, *all* spaces should have an entry with a zero or other digit entered.

ANT orients the subject's head in the Frankfort Plane, instructs him to take a breath and sit as tall as possible, and applies gentle traction to the mandible. The anthropometrist positions the anthropometer on the sitting base, and brings the branch down, crushing the hair and making firm contact with the vertex.

43. *Anterior-posterior chest depth:* the depth of the chest at mesosternale level obtained with spreading caliper or anthropometer with recurved branches used as a sliding caliper. This measure is easiest to obtain from the right side of a subject seated in an erect posture. The caliper is applied over the right shoulder in a downward direction. The olive tip of the caliper branch is held at the marked mesosternale by a pinch grip of the index finger which anchors it to the site and to the thumb. The other branch is placed on the spinous process of the vertebra at the level of the mesosternale. Again, the olive tip is anchored to the site by the index finger and maintained by the thumb. The top of the wide spreading calipers rests on the anthropometrist's chest and the anthropometer, used as a sliding caliper, rests on the anthropometrist's forearms. In using the anthropometer caliper, the moving branch may be guided by pressure along the index finger and hand. Side pressure only at the tip may cause bending. The pressure is moderately light since the olive tips can penetrate tissue and cause pain when firm pressure is applied. The measurement is taken at the end of a normal expiration (end tidal).

It should be recognized that some measures such as stature and body mass exhibit diurnal variance; one is taller and lighter in the morning and shorter and heavier in the evening under normal conditions. Repeated measuring of skinfolds also tends to compress tissue. Nevertheless, within the time required to replicate the recommended series, all obtained measures should be within the tolerance limits of the plus or minus values of a "criterion anthropometrist" as indicated in Appendix 6.6.

Derived Variables

The anthropometric data assembly in the proforma in Figure 6.7 can be used to derive the following by simple subtraction:
101 chronological age (04-05)
102 sum of skinfolds (09 to 16 inclusive)
103 arm length (17-18)
104 forearm length (18-19)
105 hand length (19-20)
106 thigh length #1 (22-23)
107 thigh length #2 (08-42-23).
These derived variables can be added to the 45 listed variables.

Resolution

Although the output is voluminous, all direct and derived variables for each sample can be processed by any number of statistical packages such as the *Statistical Package for the Social Sciences* (McGraw-Hill, 1975) which can provide such descriptive output as:
1. means
2. standard deviations
3. standard errors of the means
In addition, the data assembly provides for the anthropometric derivation of the Heath-Carter Somatotype, proportionality profiles and the anthropometric fractionation of body mass discussed in the following sections.

In ascribing meaning to individual data, it is often desirable to make a comparison to a reference group, norm or control. Truly random samples are impossible to obtain for any but limited sampling frames. At best, the sampling procedures of the Canada Fitness Survey, where satellite photographs were used to select a geographically stratified sampling of 13,440 Canadian households, yield the most representative normative data for age, sex, and geographical region available anywhere in the world.

By necessity, however, this sample had a limited anthropometric battery of 15 items.

In order to provide ancillary data on a more extensive test protocol, two reference samples were chosen. Known by their computer acronyms of CANREF and COGRO, they provide reference data of non-athletically select samples as follows: CANREF: tri-university sample of men and women selected from a general education exercise class, a university residence and a non-major physical education teachers' class. A summary of mean and standard deviation values for each variable from Carter et al., 1982 is shown as Appendix 6.3; COGRO: a three-school sample from the Coquitlam School district including 939 children age 6 to 18 years old as reported by Ross et al. (1980) (Appendix 6.4).

SOMATOTYPE

A somatotype is a physique classification based on the concept of SHAPE or the outer conformation of body composition, disregarding size. There are several systems of somatotyping; however, in athletic appraisal and guidance, the Heath-Carter method is pre-eminent. It provides for both photoscopic and anthropometric derivation of a three-component rating showing the relative dominance of –
1. endomorphy, or relative fatness
2. mesomorphy, or relative musculoskeletal robustness
3. ectomorphy, or relative linearity or "stretched-outness".

Each component is identified in sequence, endomorphy-mesomorphy-ectomorphy. With the popularization of the anthropometric derivation, the components are expressed to the nearest one-tenth rating, e.g., 1.4 – 6.0 – 3.2, an ectomorphic mesomorph, or ectomesomorph.

The method is described in detail by Carter (1980) and computer programs are available for derivation, plotting and analyses (S.P. Aubry, and J.E.L. Carter, PROSMAN Computer Programs for Somatotype Analysis, San Diego State University, San Diego, 1980).

The usual procedure is to describe the somatotypes in a sample by using mean and standard deviations of each component and to display the distribution on a bi-dimensional somatochart as shown in Figures 6.14 and 6.15. Extensive reports of somatotypes of athletes are available in the

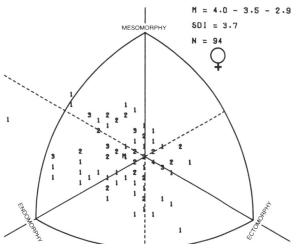

Fig. 6.14　Somatotype distribution of CANREF females.

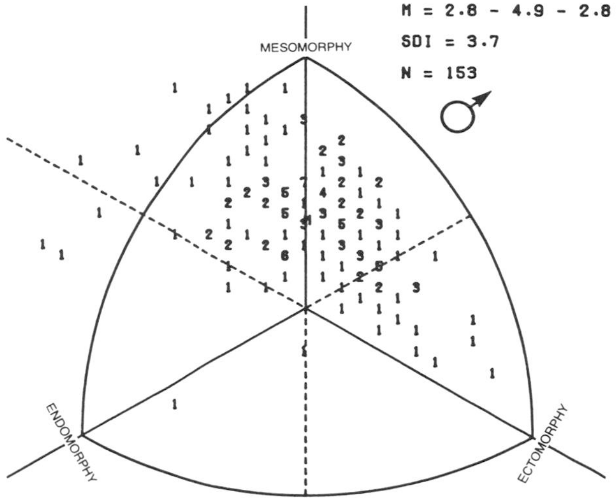

Fig. 6.15　Somatotype distribution of CANREF males.

literature. Of particular interest are a review paper on the somatotypes of female athletes by Carter (1981), the summary of adult male and female somatotype norms for Canadians aged 15 to 69, based on 13,599 participants in the YMCA-LIFE Program by Bailey et al. (1982), and the Montreal Olympic Games summaries by Carter et al. (1982).

It is not usually meaningful to analyze individual components as variables since this destroys the essential quality of "dominance" and the relationship of components in the individual subject.

In order to preserve these essential relationships in analysis, two approaches are used:

1. *Bi-dimensional analysis* of somatotype dispersion distances, or distances in Y-units between somato*plots* or plots of the 3-component somatotype as an X-Y grid where the ratio of X to Y units is 3:1 and $X = III - 1$ and $Y = 2II - (III + I)$. In this system for coordinates X1, Y1, and X2, Y2 somatotype dispersion distance

$$SDD = \sqrt{3(X1 - X2)^2 + (Y1 - Y2)^2}$$

2. *Tri-dimensional analysis* of somatotype attitudinal distances in component units when the somatotype is oriented in an X, Y, Z coordinate system. In this system, the distance between somato*points* (A and B) somatotype attitudinal distance is

$$SAD = \sqrt{(IA - IB)^2 + (IIA - IIB)^2 + (IIIA - IIIB)^2}$$

In both analytic systems, the somatotype may be calculated by a chart method or appropriate algorithms. The calculations are as follows (with variables used indicated by their Proforma number — see Figure 6.7).

Endomorphy

$$I = -0.7182 + 0.1451(X) - 0.00068(X^2) + 0.0000014(X^3)$$

where X is the sum of skinfolds #9, #10, #13. The value routinely should be height corrected by multiplying by 170.18/#08.

Mesomorphy

$$II = [0.858\#40 + 0.601\#41 + (0.188(\#27 - \#9/10)) \\ + (0.161(\#34 - \#16/10))] - (0.131\#08) + 4.50$$

Ectomorphy

$$III = 0.732(\#08/\sqrt[3]{\#07}) - 28.58$$

If $\#08/\sqrt[3]{\#07} < 40.75$ but > 38.28, then $II = 0.463(\#08/\sqrt[3]{\#07}) - 17.63$; if $\#08/\sqrt[3]{\#07} \leq 38.25$ a minimal rating of 0.1 is assigned. Note $\#08/\sqrt[3]{\#07}$ is the reciprocal of the ponderal index.

Analytic tactics and strategies are discussed in a paper entitled "Advances in somatotype methodology and analysis" by Carter et al. (1983), extensive data for athletes are presented in the literature, and large sampling norms will be available both from the Canada Fitness Survey using a specified method to estimate Heath-Carter somatotypes and from the YMCA-LIFE program report by Bailey, Carter, and Mirwald (1982).

Somatotyping is a valuable technique. It is used extensively in describing the shape characteristics of athletes. It is *not by itself a prognosticator of performance*, however, since size or other structural or functional characteristics may be operative, in addition to the myriad of other factors contributing to athletic success.

PROPORTIONALITY

Middle distance runners tend to be long in the legs and arms, short in the trunk and narrow in the hips. "Long", "short" and "narrow" are subjective evaluations based on some kind of metaphorical model of a human.

The Phantom stratagem for proportionality assessment designed by Ross and Wilson (1974), updated by Ross and Ward (1982), makes use of a single, arbitrary, unisex reference human where sizes (p) and standard deviations (s) are specified as indicated in Appendix 6.5.

The following general formula is used to translate raw scores into Phantom z-values.

$$z = \frac{1}{s}\left[v\left(\frac{170\cdot18}{h}\right)^d - p \right]$$

where:

z   is a Phantom z-value
s   is a specified Phantom standard deviation for variable v
v   is the obtained measure of variable v
170.18   is the Phantom stature constant
h   is the obtained stature
d   is the dimensional exponent. In the geometrical similarity system d is: 1 for all lengths, breadths, girths, and skinfold thicknesses; 2 for all areas; 3 for mass or volume of the whole body or any part
p   is the specified Phantom value for variable v.

The general formula has the effect of geometrically adjusting all measures to a common stature, much as achieved by changing focal lengths on a slide projector.

The d values described above are for geometrical scaling. In special circumstances other similarity systems as defined by Ross et al. (1980) may be used. It is also possible to use d values which are sample-specific. In addition, variables other than stature can be used as the scaling standard.

A z-value of 0.0 indicates variable v has the same proportion as the Phantom; a z-value greater than 0.0 indicates that the variable is proportionally larger; a negative value indicates it is proportionally smaller. Z-values can be subtracted to show differences or treated statistically as one would any standard score.

A proportionality profile, using the anthropometric proforma data in Figure 6.7, provides a rapid means of assessing a pattern. As shown in Figure 6.16, the difference between CANREF males and females can be ascertained directly when plotted on a Phantom grid. Significance may be inferred by showing bars set at two standard errors of estimates or testing for significance by usual statistical procedures.

BODY COMPOSITION

The use of skinfold prediction formulae based on densitometric validation criteria to infer "fat" content of the human body is often inappropriate

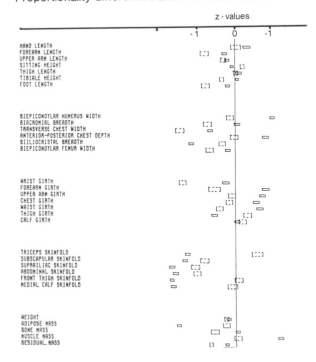

Fig. 6.16 Proportionality profiles for CANREF males and females. Broken line boxes set at 1.0 standard error from mean z-values for females. Solid line boxes set similarly for males. Non-overlapping is an inspectional test for significance of difference at approximately the five percent probability level.

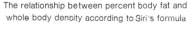

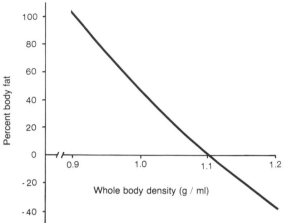

Fig. 6.17 Density assumptions and implications (Martin and Drinkwater).

resent the line of best fit, they have constants which assure negative values are not predicted. However, multiplying a sum of skinfold by a constant and adding another gives the investigator no additional information other than the use of the simple sum of the skinfolds. Similarly, density values are meaningful in themselves, and nothing further is gained by transformation to percent fat.

Skinfold caliper data expressed as a simple sum of the sites recommended in the proforma are useful in monitoring dietary and training influences. Moreover, the individual sites show the individual external adipose tissue patterning which, in itself, is of research interest since this seems to have predictable individual characteristics in subsequent gain or loss in body mass.

Recent cadaver dissection studies have shown that some lower extremity sites have higher relationships with total dissectable adiposity than some of the more popular upper body sites used in prediction formulae. The eight sites in the proforma provide for a minimum sampling of the body sites and are recommended in routine assessment.

for appraisal in athletes.

The difficulty arises in having to accept the necessary assumption that the human body may be conceived of as a two-compartment model with known densities of the fat and non-fat compartments. As shown in Figure 6.17, the strategy is to measure whole body density corrected for lung and visceral gas volumes and then infer fat percentage from density values. For example, in the popular formula by Siri (1961), arbitrarily assigned density values of 0.900 g·ml^{-1} to the "fat" portion and 1.100 g·ml^{-1} to the non-fat portion are used to indicate 100% fat and 0% fat respectively. When the assumptions are tenable, percent fat can be inferred from body density as illustrated in Figure 6.17.

The assigned density of 1.1000 g·ml^{-1} for the non-fat compartment is grossly violated by some athletes who have denser bone and muscle and a larger proportion of these in the non-fat portion than average. Thus, obtained whole body densities higher than 1.1000 would indicate "negative fat". Eight out of 22 members of the Edmonton Eskimo professional football team as reported by Adams et al. (1981, 1982) had density values in this range. This is not an artifact of measurement, since other investigators have found similar density values in extreme ectomesomorphic subjects.

Because the conventional skinfold prediction formulae based on such densitometric criteria rep-

Anthropometric Fractionation of Body Mass

If one assumes adiposity varies as the skinfolds, bone mass as the bone breadths, muscle mass as the skinfold thickness corrected girths, and the residual mass (organs, viscera, fluids) as the size of the thorax, a four-way fractionation of body mass is feasible, as discussed by Drinkwater and Ross (1980) and most recently described by Ross et al. (1981). The so called "Drinkwater tactic" is based on the premise that the sum of Phantom z-values for each fraction will vary as the fractional mass of the Phantom.

The Phantom specification for the anthropometric fractionation of body mass is illustrated in Figure 6.18. The "fat mass", for example, is based on the premise that it deviates from the Phantom as the deviation of the indicator variables, that is, the skinfold thicknesses.

If, for example, the mean of the z-values for any given number of skinfolds was $-1.0z$, we should expect the fat mass to be one standard deviation (S) less than the Phantom fat mass (P). The given Phantom P and S values are 12.13 and 3.25 kg. Therefore, $-1.0z$ in the mean skinfolds would be $12.13 - 3.25 = 8.88$ kg. This value item then would have to be rescaled to the subject's actual stature as follows:

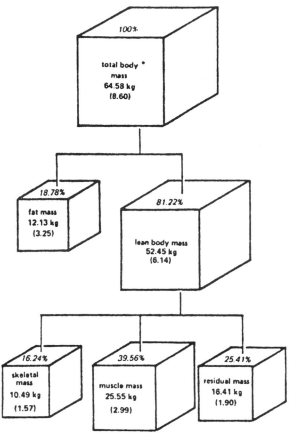

Fig. 6.18　Fractionation of body mass chart.

$$[8.88/(170.18/h)^3]$$

As discussed in the original paper, the tactic employs the above principles in the following general formula for subjects of variables selected to yield estimates of fat, bone, muscle and residual masses.

$$M = \frac{(\bar{Z} \times S) + P}{\left(\dfrac{170.18}{h}\right)^d}$$

where:

M is the estimated fractional mass

$\bar{Z}$ is the mean Phantom z-value calculated from the selected subset of variables

P and S are Phantom values and their standard deviations for the fractional masses

h is the subject's obtained stature

d is a dimensional exponent which has the value 3 in this application.

The main advantages of the four-way fractionation of body mass are:

1. It estimates the muscle-mass which is related to strength and is the relevant tissue for appraisal of metabolic events.

2. The total of the estimated fractions must approximate the total obtained body mass under normal conditions of hydration (within about 5%) and this serves as an internal validity criterion.

3. Differences in fat, muscle, bone, and residual mass among individuals and samples can be summarized for easy interpretation as shown in Figure 6.19 for the CANREF samples (Ross et al., 1981).

It is the nature of science to build new models from ruined structures. The four-way fractionation of body mass avoids some of the pitfalls of the two-component model. However, it, too, must be thought of as a practical procedure which will, in turn, give way to a more sophisticated model. Undoubtedly, the concept of "fat" will be replaced by an anatomical entity, "the dissectable adipose tissue mass," which has internal and external portions which are probably not deducible as a simple function of skinfold thicknesses. The model will be somewhat more elaborate. More accurate regional assessment of muscle and bone will be available with subsequent anatomical studies buttressed with CAT scanning as body composition becomes a focus for research enterprise. These studies will lead to more definitive work on the relationship of strength, metabolic events and performance to the relevant tissue masses. Herein lies the common ground for theorists, experimenters, and practitioners.

Densitometry

Densitometry is a technique for the assessment of total body density. Density has often been used as a means of estimating "fat" and "fat-free" masses (Behnke, 1942; Siri, 1961). Whilst nothing is achieved by forcing density values into percent fat estimates, density itself is an important parameter since it is a quotient of two of the three basic human structural parameters, viz. stature, body mass and body volume.

A number of indirect methods are available for the assessment of body density. This manual, however, will deal with only two methods, both of which assess total body volume: hydrostatic weighing, and volume displacement using a body volumeter.

Figure 6.20 illustrates a system capable of providing simultaneous direct measurements of hydrostatic weight and volume displacement. Concurrently, residual lung volumes (which are subtracted to give a net body volume) are obtained using a closed-circuit nitrogen washout technique.

Basic density measuring systems incorporate either an underwater weighing device or a manometer for measuring displaced water. In either situation apparatus for measuring residual volume is essential. The use of a dual system in the Kinanthropometry Laboratory at Simon Fraser University permits simultaneous determinations of body volume and thus provides cross-validation of results.

The complete protocol will be outlined and, should only one of the volume techniques be used, the directions pertaining to the other can be ignored.

The subject is weighed in air using a weighing scale, calibrated from 0-150,000 g, damped to reduce oscillations below 20 g stability. The subject should be wet during this weighing, so should be asked to rinse in a shower prior to measurement. This also assists in the removal of any extraneous body dirt or grease.

A number of readings must be taken before commencing testing in the tank. These are: barometric pressure, tank water temperature, laboratory room temperature, initial manometer level, and baseline readings for the nitrogen analyzer and weight transducer on the four-channel

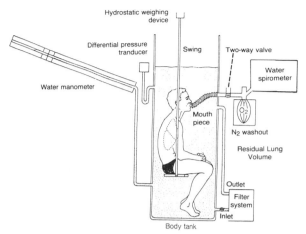

Fig. 6.20 Simultaneous hydrostatic weighing and water displacement volumeter.

recorder.

Once the preliminary baseline readings have been taken and a volume of oxygen approximating the subject's inspiratory capacity (3-4 ℓ; the precise volume must be measured using the attached spirometer) has been injected into the bag-in-box system, the subject gets into the tank. The subject inserts the mouthpiece and the swing is adjusted so that the seated subject is immersed to neck level.

Following several minutes of quiescent breathing of room air through the two-way valve (see Figure 6.20), the swing is further lowered until the top of the subject's head is 10-15 cm below the

---

FRACTIONATED BODY MASS IN MALE AND FEMALE UNIVERSITY STUDENTS SHOWING
DEVIATIONS FROM UNISEX REFERENCE HUMAN OR PHANTOM

| Tissue masses | MALES (n - 152) | | | | | FEMALES (n - 94) | | | | |
| | PHANTOM | | DERIVED MASSES | | | PHANTOM | | DERIVED MASSES | | |
	$\bar{z}$	sd	$\bar{x}$	sd	%	$\bar{z}$	sd	$\bar{x}$	sd	%
Adipose	− 1.61	0.73	7.92	2.76	10.96	− 0.29	0.93	10.38	2.98	18.04
Bone	0.06	0.79	12.20	1.58	16.88	− 0.63	0.78	8.76	1.20	15.22
Muscle	1.24	0.76	33.78	3.93	46.75	0.32	0.74	24.48	2.64	42.54
Residual	− 0.26	0.62	18.36	2.03	25.41	− 0.71	0.58	13.92	1.50	24.19
Predicted mass, (p)			72.26					57.54		
Obtained mass, (o)			72.35					57.48		
Difference (p-o), (d)			− 0.09					0.06		
Percent error 100, (d/o)			0.12%					0.10%		

Fig. 6.19 CANREF fractionation summary.

surface of the water. The subject is then specifically directed to inhale and exhale three times, the tester audibly calling the rate, and to hold what is left of his breath at the end of the third exhalation, which should be maximal. Underwater weight and manometer level readings are taken at this point and the two-way valve is then switched over so that the subject's next inhalation will be from the bag-in-box system. The subject is then coached to take 5 to 8 maximal inspiratory capacity breaths, to facilitate rapid nitrogen equilibration.

Once the nitrogen value has re-stabilized, the two-way valve is switched back to room air. The subject can then take the mouthpiece out and exit from the tank. Baseline values for volume and weight are checked, the bag-in-box system is flushed with pure oxygen and 3 to 4 litres of oxygen are injected into the bag in readiness for the second trial.

The complete procedure is repeated twice to obtain triplicate measures.

Using the following formula, residual lung volume can be calculated. This must then be corrected to BTPS before its use in the formula for calculating density:

$$R.V. = \left[\frac{(BV + DSa)\ (Cb)}{(Ca - Cb)} - DSb \right] \times BTPS$$

where:

BV   = volume (ml) of oxygen in bag of bag-box calculated from the difference between the two spirometer readings.

DSa   = volume (ml) of space from top of bag of bag-box to the two-way valve, i.e., tube deadspace.

Cb   = nitrogen concentration at equilibration (%).

DSb   = volume of deadspace from two-way valve to subject.

Ca   = initial nitrogen concentration (%). (At maximal expiration.)

BTPS   = Body Temperature Pressure Saturation conversion factor. (See Appendix 6.2.)

It is customary to subtract a constant of 100 ml (BTPS) for estimated gastro-intestinal volume of gas. This value is presumably when the subject is in a post-absorptive state, and is applied regardless of the size of the subject. To be consistent with other scaling, the value could be adjusted for stature by multiplying by $(170.18/\text{height})^3$. Very limited cadaver data suggest that this value of 100 ml may be too low. However, when evidence

is lacking, adherence to convention assures systematic error in the results.

Body volume can then be calculated on the basic principle of dividing mass by volume.

$$\text{Density} = \frac{\text{Weight in Air}}{\text{Volume} - (\text{Residual Volume} + \text{G.I. gas})}$$

A correction for the density of the water in the tank must be made when calculating volume from hydrostatic weighing. The equation used in this instance is:

$$\text{Density} = \frac{\text{Weight in Air}}{\dfrac{W(air) - W(water)}{\text{Density(water)}} - (R.V. + G.I.\ gas)}$$

The volume in the tank is immaterial in the underwater weighing procedure. However, in the displacement procedure, the smaller the volume consistent with subject comfort the better.

Safety. One must recognize any small volume of water with heavy usage requires fastidious cleanliness. Water treatment procedures are essential, including heating, circulation, filtration and approved disinfectant agents similar to those prescribed for swimming pools under the various provincial and municipal codes. Ensuring that all laboratory electronic equipment, lighting, pumps, hoists and heating systems are properly grounded is a basic, yet often overlooked, precaution.

To facilitate accurate measurement, the subject should be twelve hours post-absorptive. The subject should be weighed nude (preferably) or with minimal clothing (the weight of which should be measured and adjusted for). He should be asked to remove any entrapped air from the body surface upon submerging and required to wear a noseclip. The subject should be allowed to practise the measuring maneuver and then at least three measurement trials should be undertaken to ensure full exhalation and hence minimal weight in the water.

Comprehensive Compositional Assessment

Somatotype, density, proportionality profiles and the fractionation of body mass should provide a comprehensive picture of the body composition of an athlete. For example a 1 - 7.5 - 3, is an extreme ectomesomorph, the 7.5 indicating extreme musculo-skeletal robustness, which may be reflected in a density value as high as 1.20 $g \cdot ml^{-1}$ (negative fat if one is naïve enough to use current assumptions). This will be reflected in the high z-values for skinfold-corrected muscle girth and bone breadth values. The status of body composition may also be summarized by the fractionation procedure which may show this subject's body mass to be comprised of 5% adiposity, 20% bone, 50% muscle and 25% residual.

MATURATION

The earliest maturing 12-year-old girl in grade six is physiologically as old as the latest maturing first year university male student. Generally, girls mature earlier than boys. The average girl has her peak stature velocity during her adolescent growth spurt about age 12, whereas the average boy has his about age 14. Because the peak stature velocity may occur as much as two years earlier or later than the average, a six-year difference in the event between the early maturing girl and later maturing boy is quite possible.

Maturity Events

Some indication of the maturity status of a young athlete can be inferred from longitudinal stature data.

Tri-dimensional Computer Graphics in Growth Curve Analysis

The individual velocity curves generated by a computer and displayed tri-dimensionally are as discussed by Leahy et al. (1980). As shown in Figure 6.21, individual curves for a sample may be ordered for relative maturity by the shape characteristics. This kind of monitoring and display of a whole national team, such as gymnasts, would be invaluable. It avoids complex analyses, yet permits identification of individual characteristics at any time in the context of the sample pattern. The interactive possibilities of the computer in rotating axes and scaling provides many options. The curve, however, is only as good as the precision and frequency of the data input (see sections on *Longitudinal Evaluation* and *Precision and Accuracy*).

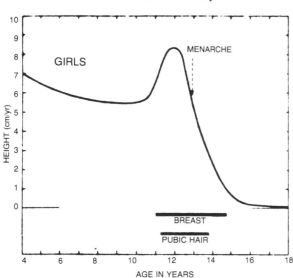

MATURITY EVENTS IN GIRLS

Peak height velocity in girls occurs about twelve years of age. Usually the first physical sign of adolescence is noted in breast budding which occurs slightly after the onset of the growth spurt. Shortly thereafter, pubic hair begins to grow. Menarche or the onset of menstruation comes rather late in the growth spurt, occurring after peak height velocity is achieved. The whole sequence of events, however, may normally occur two or even more years earlier or later than average. Ross et al. (1977)

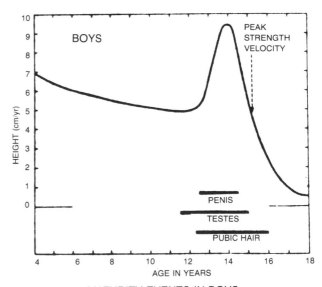

MATURITY EVENTS IN BOYS

The adolescent growth spurt in boys is more intense than in girls and on the average it occurs about two years later. Growth of the testes, pubic hair and penis are related to the maturation process. Peak strength velocity comes a year or so after peak height velocity. Thus, there is a pronounced late gain in strength characteristic of the male growth pattern. The whole developmental sequence may occur two or more years earlier or later than average. Thus, early maturing boys may have as much as a four-year physiological advantage over their later maturing peers. Eventually, however, the late maturers will catch up when they experience their growth spurt. Ross et al. (1977)

STANDING HEIGHT VELOCITY

SASKATCHEWAN BOYS
Age 7 to 16 years on X axis, cm per
year on Y axis, and subjects on Z axis.

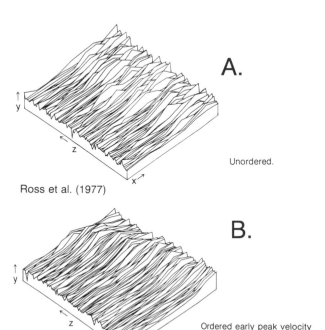

A.

Unordered.

Ross et al. (1977)

B.

Ordered early peak velocity
point in background,
late in foreground.

Fig. 6.21 Tri-dimensional graph of 100 boys from Saskatchewan Growth Study. (Leahy et al., 1980)

Skeletal Age

In the absence of longitudinal stature data and ancillary evidence of secondary sex characteristics and age of menarche, a rating of a *left* hand and wrist radiograph is the definitive assessment. However, radiographic techniques requiring even minimal exposure to X-rays is usually *not* justified unless it is under medical guidance and radiographic evidence is justified on clinical grounds. In the United Kingdom, a simple guideline for research purposes is to permit one radiograph per lifetime. In Canada, the use of X-rays for research and diagnostic purposes is a medical prerogative and, presumably, university research enterprise is appropriately monitored by ethics committees.

When appropriate, the radiographic technique should be according to the IBP specification (Weiner and Lourie, 1981). Several methods of assessment have been shown to provide reliable estimates of skeletal age. Because of the ease of scrutiny of the decision-making processes, which involve bone-specific rating, the method of choice is the T-W II of Tanner-Whitehouse (1975).

A criterion set of 113 radiographs is used at the Institute of Child Health, University of London, as a standard for determining competence. (Copies are presently at SFU.) The time involvement for a perceptive trainee is roughly that of a one-semester 3-hour-per-week course, or about sixty hours including preliminary reading and orientation. Introduction to the method in kinanthropometry and pediatric courses involving half-a-dozen rating attempts is not adequate for individual diagnostic purposes.

In interpreting skeletal age, the total bone rating is related to norms. In the T-W method the norms are based on British children who were, at the time, not as mature as upper middle-class children in Cleveland, who are also used as norms. Thus, as for any cross-sectional comparisons, the interpretation of norms must be in relation to the sample supplying the basic data.

It should be recognized that radiographs are portable data. They can easily be copied and sent to several independent raters. Ideally, this should be done, particularly when the investigators have inadequate experience and need corroborative estimates.

Menarche

"Men-ar-kee" or the *onset of the first menstrual flow* (even though subsequently irregular), is a recognized biological benchmark.

Since 1800, there has been a secular trend toward earlier age of menarche. From around 17 in the 1770's, it has progressively declined in many countries to about 12.5 to 13.0 years with a plateauing in this range noted in recent years.

Three methods are used to estimate menarche. The best, most reliable, is to include the item as part of a longitudinal appraisal. Athletes, coaches and parents should alert girls that the age of menarche is an important developmental event which should be recorded. When the date occurs, it can be noted routinely. Normative values can be established by the status-quo method. This involves asking a large sample of girls age 8 to 18 two questions: (1) date of birth; (2) have you yet had your first menstrual flow, first period? From the age and yes/no answers it is possible by logits and probits to calculate mean and standard deviation age of menarche values. The third method appropriate for individual and sampling studies is the recall method.

In samples of grade 12 students and university women, with careful interviewing technique, the recall may be as high as 80 percent certain or fairly certain. Because athletes have memorable dates of competition, recall may be enhanced by association. Although some males are able to elicit the information, a woman who is perceived by the girls as a "medical person", "scientist" or "counsellor" seems to have an advantage.

Announcing that the question will be asked a day or so ahead of time permits the respondents to do some reflective thinking. A simple questionnaire asks the respondents if they have experienced menarche (explained as the first menstrual flow) yes or no. If yes, they are asked to indicate the year and month. In aiding the respondent to recall, discussion is focussed on associated events. Typical questions by the investigator might include — What grade were you in at the time? . . . was it Spring or Fall? . . . during summer vacations? . . . was it when you started back to school? . . . was it around Christmas? . . . was it during a particular exam period? . . . was it close to or during some competitive event when the date is known?

After the decision is made, the investigator can have the respondent evaluate her recall as 0 = not yet; 1 = certain; 2 = fairly certain; 3 = approximate; 4 = uncertain; 5 = unwilling to respond.

In calculating age of menarche from month estimate, the 15th day of the month can be used as a specific day for use of decimal fraction of years. Thus, differences in age of menarche of less than 0.1 year are trivial.

While there is a secular trend to earlier maturation, Malina (1982a, 1982b) noted in sports where girls were required to move their body mass, like gymnastics and track and field, elite female athletes tend to be *late* maturers. Ross et al. (1977) reported delayed menarche in elite figure skaters and normal menarche in alpine skiers. The above data and a sample of all of the participants in the 1977 Canadian Synchronized Swimming Championships and three non-athletically select samples were summarized by Ross and Ward (1980) and augmented by a recent report by Marker (1981).

There is controversy in the literature whether heavy training resulting in a lean physique is related to delayed maturation, or if the qualities of smallness and leanness are selective factors in certain sports.

The question appears moot since experimental data are generally not available. Beunen (1976) in assessing unrelated girls 11 to 13 years old found early maturers were taller and had better equilibrium than average or late maturers. Only slight differences were found among maturity levels at ages 14 and 16. However, at age 16 to 18, the late-maturing girls always obtained better results than their average or early-maturing peers. The phenomenon might well be related to the effective muscle/body mass relationship.

Unsubstantiated observations suggest heavy training may be a causal factor in delayed maturation, since female athletes forced into inactivity by injury or other causes sometimes show accelerated maturation. Again, evidence is lacking for a definitive statement.

Until recently it was not known if there is a beneficial or deleterious effect from delayed maturation. A comprehensive report at the 'Women in Sport' Congress in Rome by Marker (1981) showed no apparent harmful effect of delayed menarche or sport amenorrhea (temporary suspension of menstruation) and no later gynaecological difficulties or parturition problems compared to non-athletic women. Medical records favouring the athletic sample may simply be a reflection of better health status rather than any specific training effect.

The long-term monitoring of athletes can do much to dispel fantasy and myths which restricted females from competitive athletics for many years.

Genitalia Assessment

The secondary sex characteristics can be used as a simple ancillary method of rating maturational development. The ratings can be made in the course of a medical, anthropometric, or densitometric protocol affording a view of the nude subject. Somatotype photographs of the nude subject are an alternative, though particular care must be taken when using this method. The subject should be masked when photographed, and control exercised on photographic processing as well as on the filing and recording systems.

Ethical and cultural factors enter into the decision to rate pubic hair, genital and breast development.

In situations where such data is needed for full maturity appraisal, but ethical or cultural factors intervene, a compromise procedure is to have the subject make a self-rating in private.

A six-point scale is used with "1" indicating a prepubescent stage and "6" adult conformation, as shown in the line drawings and descriptions in Figures 6.22, 6.23, 6.24, and 6.25.

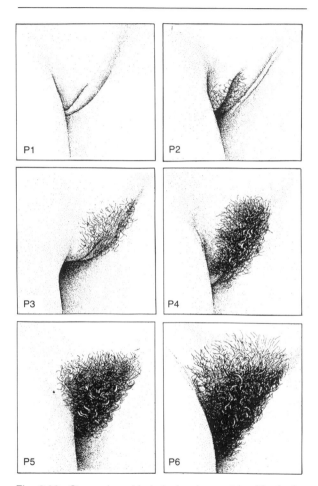

Fig. 6.22 Stages in pubic hair development in girls. In the development of pubic hair, six stages can be distinguished:
P1 — no growth of pubic hair.
P2 — initial, scarcely pigmented hair, especially along the labia (not visible on black-white photographs).
P3 — sparse dark, visibly pigmented, curly pubic hair on labia.
P4 — hair 'adult' in type, but not in extent.
P5 — lateral spreading; type and spread of hair — adult.
P6 — further extension laterally, upwards, or disperse (apparently occurs in only 10% of women).

Redrawn, with permission, from *Growth Diagrams 1965*, by J.C. Van Wieringen, F. Wafelbakker, H.P. Verbrugge, J.H. De Haas, Nederlands Instituut voor Praeventieve Gezondheidszorg TNO. Wolters-Noordhoff Publishing, Groningen, 1971.

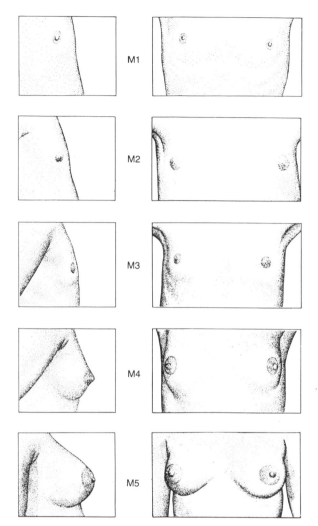

Fig. 6.23 Stages in breast development in girls. The development of the mammae can be divided into five stages:
M1 — only the nipple is raised above the level of the breast, as in the child.
M2 — budding stage: bud-shaped elevation of the areola. On palpation, a fairly hard 'button' can be felt, disc- or cherry-shaped. Areola increased in diameter and surrounding area slightly elevated.
M3 — further elevation of the mammae. Areolar diameter increased further. Shape of mammae now visibly feminine.
M4 — increasing fat deposits. The areola forms a secondary elevation above that of the breast. This secondary mound apparently occurs in roughly half of all girls, and in some cases persists in adulthood.
M5 — adult stage. The areola (usually) subsides to the level of the breast and is strongly pigmented.

Redrawn, with permission, from *Growth Diagrams 1965*, by J.C. Van Wieringen, F. Wafelbakker, H.P. Verbrugge, J.H. De Haas, Nederlands Instituut voor Praeventieve Gezondheidszorg TNO. Wolters-Noordhoff Publishing, Groningen, 1971.

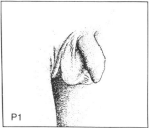
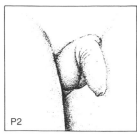
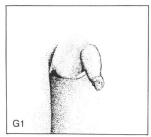
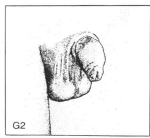

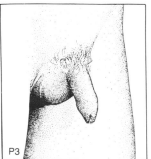
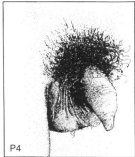
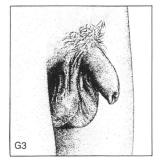
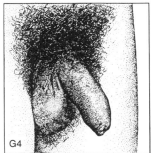

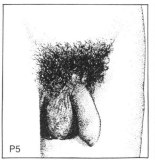
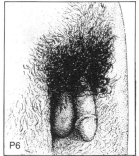
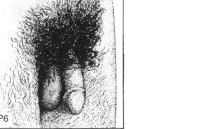
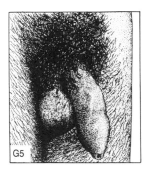

Fig. 6.24 Stages in pubic hair development in boys. As in girls, development of pubic hair can be divided into six stages.

P1 — no growth of pubic hair, i.e. hair in pubic area no different from that on the rest of the abdomen.

P2 — slightly pigmented, longer, straight hair, often still downy; usually at base of penis, sometimes on scrotum. Stage 2 is difficult to photograph.

P3 — dark, definitely pigmented, curly pubic hair around base of penis. Stage 3 can be photographed.

P4 — pubic hair definitely adult in type, but not in extent (no further than inguinal fold).

P5 — spread to medial surface of thighs, but not upwards.

P6 — hair spreads along linea alba (supposed to occur in 80% of men).

Redrawn, with permission, from *Growth Diagrams 1965*, by J.C. Van Wieringen, F. Wafelbakker, H.P. Verbrugge, J.H. De Haas, Nederlands Instituut voor Praeventieve Gezondheidszorg TNO. Wolters-Noordhoff Publishing, Groningen, 1971.

Fig. 6.25 Stages of genital development in boys. The development of the external genitalia can be differentiated in five stages.

G1 — testes, scrotum and penis are the same size and shape as in the young child.

G2 — enlargement of scrotum and testes. The skin of the scrotum becomes redder, thinner and wrinkled. Penis no larger or scarcely so.

G3 — enlargement of the penis, especially in length; further enlargement of testes; descent of scrotum.

G4 — continued enlargement of the penis and sculpturing of the glans. Increased pigmentation of the scrotum. This stage is sometimes best described as 'not quite adult'.

G5 — adult stage. Scrotum ample, penis reaching nearly to bottom of scrotum.

Redrawn, with permission, from *Growth Diagrams 1965*, by J.C. Van Wieringen, F. Wafelbakker, H.P. Verbrugge, J.H. De Haas, Nederlands Instituut voor Praeventieve Gezondheidszorg TNO. Wolters-Noordhoff Publishing, Groningen, 1971.

Prediction of Adult Stature

By analysis of data derived from a sufficient number of children measured longitudinally, it becomes possible to say what percentage of their final adult height has been achieved at any given age, and thus to produce a table which will predict with some accuracy the future height of an individual from measurements taken in childhood (Table 6.1).

The predictive value of such a table is nil at birth, for the birth length, like the birth weight, is considerably influenced by the environment of the foetus in the womb. For example, a baby, ultimately destined by its genetic make-up to be tall, may measure relatively little at birth if it is premature, one of a multiple birth, or born to a young mother.

By the second birthday, however, the child has joined the genetic curve which basically determines his height, and predictions become reasonable.

From the age of three years to the age of 8 years for girls and 10 years for boys, the predictive reliability is quite high.

After that time, the percentages apply only to girls and boys who have peak stature velocities at 12 and 14 years respectively. The use of other percentile standards, and skeletal age, with some expectancy of precision in prediction, is discussed by Tanner (1978).

Table 6.1   Percentage of mature height attained at different ages.

CHRONOLOGICAL AGE	PERCENTAGE OF EVENTUAL HEIGHT	
(years)	Boys	Girls
1	42.2	44.7
2	49.5	52.8
3	53.8	57.0
4	58.0	61.8
5	61.8	66.2
6	65.2	70.3
7	69.0	74.0
8	72.0	77.5
9	75.0	80.7
10	78.0	84.4
11	81.1	88.4
12	84.2	92.9
13	87.3	96.5
14	91.5	98.3
15	96.1	99.1
16	98.3	99.6
17	99.3	100.0
18	99.8	100.0

(Bayley, N. 1954)

SIZE AND PERFORMANCE EXPECTATION

The comment that a particular athlete is good for his or her size implies an appreciation of human dimensionality. However, such impressions are imprecise and are based on subjective judgments which often defy meaningful analysis.

Allometry

Huxley's general allometric equation $Y = aX^b$ or its log-log identity, $\log Y = \log a + b \log X$, provides a simple method for dimensional scaling and comparison with geometrical and other similarity systems as discussed by Ross et al. (1980a).

In these equations, X is usually a structural variable, mass or stature, and Y is a functional variable such as strength, maximal aerobic or anaerobic power, or any other performance measure.

The obtained b-values are then compared to theoretical expectancy for a given similarity system. The most common comparison is to that of a geometrical system where *size and shape are constant*. Departures thus are regarded as violations of the basic assumption.

If, indeed, shape and composition were constant, the theory holds that all measures increase as a function of L in length as follows:

as L for all linear measures such as length, breadths, girths and skinfold thickness

L^2 for all *areas*, cross-section of bone and muscle (strength) or surface area of the body

L^3 for all *volumes* and *masses* for the total body or any of its parts.

It also follows in this theoretical system that force has the same dimensions as *strength* L^2 and, from Newton's second law (that $F(L^2) \propto$ mass (L^3) times acceleration (LT^{-2})), that time (T) has the dimension (L).

Strength

Theoretically, we should expect strength proportional to body mass to be a function of mass to the power two-thirds (0.667). This was found to hold true for the performance in weight lifting per upper limit of the weight classification for Olympic champion performances for each Olympiad 1928 to 1976, i.e. mean exponent 0.692 (0.052) as reported by Ross et al. (1980).

Growing children, however, do not grow as geometrical entities. They change in shape and composition. In general, they become more linear, less boney, and more muscular with increasing age.

The strength expectancy of mass to 0.667 is greatly exceeded by values in the longitudinal study for boys age 6 to 18 years in Saskatchewan of 1.65 for five cable tension tests and 1.16 in Medford boys for eleven cable tension strength tests as well as 1.28, 1.03, and 1.93 for right grip, pull-ups and parallel bar dips reported by Ross et al. (1978) and Ross and Corlett (1980). Thus, as boys increase in size, they grow in strength performance greater than geometrical expectancy. Until the post-pubescent period, girls presumably have a similar dimensional increase, although, as discussed by Ross and Ward (1981), the proportional increase in upper arm girth of girls is far exceeded by boys, suggesting an increasing sexual dimorphism in upper body strength.

Oxygen Uptake

Dimensionality in matters of maximal oxygen uptake is poorly understood. Three examples serve to illustrate: (1) in Sweden, growing Olympic swimmers trained harder than ever before in their lives. As the team physician reported in the Bisham Abbey Pediatric Work Physiology Symposium, they improved in swim time and all the usual physiological parameters but, in terms of maximal oxygen uptake, they declined in $ml \cdot kg^{-1} \cdot min^{-1}$. (2) Canadian figure skaters were told to add aerobic training to achieve stamina in freeskating. They did. Running improved, they achieved greater stamina in skating, yet on retest six months later they found they had declined in predicted maximal aerobic power expressed in $ml \cdot kg^{-1} \cdot min^{-1}$. (3) Calculation using data from 23 studies reported in the literature showed the same phenomenon in 15 of them.

Children do not increase in maximal oxygen uptake according to the increase in body mass or to the geometric expectancy of stature squared or mass to the power two-thirds.

In Saskatchewan boys, Bailey (1978) reported mean values of maximal oxygen uptake in 51 boys studied longitudinally, age 8 to 15 years, as 2.46 for stature and 0.89 for body mass.

If one wishes to use these actually determined dimensions to dissociate size and growth effects, the following formulae proposed by Ross (1978) can be used:

$$\dot{V}O_2 \text{ max rel } h = (\dot{V}O_2 \, \ell \cdot min^{-1} \cdot h^{-2.46}) \, 10^7$$

$$\dot{V}O_2 \text{ max rel } w = (\dot{V}O_2 \, \ell \cdot min^{-1} \cdot w^{0.89}) \, 1180$$

where h and w are stature and body mass and 10^7 and 1180 are constants which yield a value of 100 for mean values for the Saskatchewan sample. The interpretation is "if stature and mass had the same dimension in a given subject as the Saskatchewan boys, he would have a value of 100." Thus 100 plus or minus values indicate greater or lesser relative or size-dissociated maximal oxygen uptake values than Saskatchewan boys.

The mixed-longitudinal data in Saskatchewan girls have not yet been resolved.

It should be recognized that the Saskatchewan growth study data were collected prior to the recent fitness boom. Studies conducted when there is an increasingly enriched ambient exercise environment will have elevated b-values. Thus, it may be that experimenters will show maximal oxygen uptake approaches or even exceeds the dimension of mass to the first power. This, however, is not proof of the phenomenon that it is a function of body mass or that body mass should be the universal divisor.

Experimenters can and should report maximal oxygen uptake values as raw liters per minute. They may also report it as a ratio, using body mass as a divisor if desired. *In addition* they should report the actual log-log relationships of: (1) maximal oxygen uptake and body mass; (2) maximal oxygen uptake and stature; (3) body mass and stature. The use of the Saskatchewan formulae is optional and may be superceded whenever more extensive longitudinal evidence becomes available. Any performance and size relationship can be expressed in much the same way. When this is done, differences between samples may be minimized since performance is often size-dependent with children performing exactly to their structural characteristics.

COMPETENCY OF PERSONNEL

A kinanthropometrist should have a basic understanding of human biology, technical ability to measure, and familiarity with the following concepts used in the interpretation of data:

- Conventions in graphing.
- Construction of distance curve.
- Correction for time of measurement.
- Velocity polygon.
- Velocity histogram.
- Acceleration polygon.
- Linear regression.
- Correlation coefficients, product-moment.
- Standard error of estimate.
- Common variance and predictive index.
- Chi-square.
- Contingency and other coefficients of correlation.
- Spurious correlations, causation and circumstantial evidence.
- Inter- and intra-observer reliability, attenuation.
- Theory of error and effects on systems of measurement.
- Percentiles, t-scores, Hull scores, stanine scores, sigma scales, quartiles, ranges, tolerances.
- Descriptive statistics, mean, mode, standard deviation.
- Standard error formulae and interpretation.
- Normality, skewness, kurtosis, transformations.
- Dimensionality and similarity systems.
- Allometry and interpretation of growth and performance phenomena.
- Somatotype, somatotype categories.
- Somatochart, plotting, dispersion.
- Bi- and tri-dimensional somatotype conventions.
- Cross-sectional and longitudinal somatotype sample distribution analyses.
- Proportionality assessment.
- Metaphorical models, theoretical and prototypical models.
- Proportionality profiles and significance testing.
- Archimedes Principle and densitometry.
- Anthropometric fractionation of body mass systems.
- Rating scales and factor-point value systems (e.g. skeletal age, gymnastics, figure skating rating).
- Operations for the above on hand-held calculators.
- Computer operations for the above in addition to SPSS and BIOMED standard programs.

FEE STRUCTURE

The recommended fee schedule for kinanthropometric evaluations, per subject, is as follows:

(1) Anthropometry: triple measures by criterion anthropometrist, copy to subject. $25.00
(2) Resolution of data, with report of somatotype, proportionality profile, fractionation of body mass; related to appropriate norm base. $10.00
(3) Densitometry. $40.00
(4) Skeletal age rating: by trained rater (excluding cost of radiograph). $20.00
(5) Genitalia assessment: nude or photographic rating. . . . . $ 5.00
(6) Consultant services to establish objectivity or to initiate kinanthropometric appraisal and guidance programs. . . . . IWKG RATES

(IWGK: $300(US) per day for first two days, $150 thereafter, plus travel and accommodation. Criterion anthropometrist: $150 per day, first two days, $75 thereafter, plus travel and accommodation. Team measurement by negotiation.)

ACKNOWLEDGMENTS

The authors gratefully acknowledge the staff members of Simon Fraser University Instructional Media Center, in particular, Doris Coombes for the original drawing of the Phantom; Jaclynne Campbell for the skeletal landmarks drawing prepared for "Anthropometric concomitants of X-chromosome aneuploidies" in The Cytogenetics of the Mammalian X-Chromosome, by W.D. Ross, R. Ward, B.A. Sigmon, R.M. Leahy, edited by A.V. Sandberg, and published by Alan R. Liss, New York, 1983, and for the drawing of genitalia from photographic standards; Derek Parkin for the drawing of the volumeter and assistance in the design of the measurement proforma; and Bill Schuss for the design of the kinanthropometry logo. The authors also acknowledge the permission to redraw the genitalia standards developed by J.C. Van Wieringen, F. Wafelbakker, H.P. Verbrugge, J.H. De Haas, the Netherlands Institute for Preventive Medicine TNO, Leiden, and Wolters-Noordhoff Publishing Company, Groningen, The Netherlands, the publishers of an excellent basal reference entitled Growth Diagrams 1965 Netherlands, second national survey on 0-24-year-olds. The authors also recognize the voluntary contribution in various field trials of anthropometric techniques by the following friends and colleagues: R. Ward, N.O. Whittingham, R. Miller, A. Rapp, D.T. Drinkwater, R.M. Leahy, A.D. Martin, K. Mittleman, S. Crawford, C. Bowes, A.S. Vajda-Janyk, S.R. Brown, B. Howe.

REFERENCES

Adams, J., M. Mottola, K.M. Bagnall, K.D. McFadden. Total body fat content in a group of professional football players. *Can. J. Appl. Spt. Sc.* 7: 1, 36-40, 1982.

Adams, J., K.M. Bagnall, K.D. McFadden, M. Mottola. Body density differences between negro and caucasian professional football players. *Brit. J. Sports. Med.* 15(4) 257-260, 1981.

Bailey, D.A., W.D. Ross, R.L. Mirwald, C. Weese. Size disassociation of maximal aerobic power during growth in boys. *Pediatric Work Physiology.* J. Borms and M. Hebbelinck (eds). Karger: Basel, 11, 140-151, 1978.

Bailey, D.A., J.E.L. Carter, R.L. Mirwald. Somatotypes of Canadian men and women. *Human Biology*, 54: 4, 813-828, 1982.

Bayley, N. The accurate prediction of growth and adult height. *Mod. Prob. in Pediatrics.* 7, 234-255, 1954.

Behnke, A.R., B.G. Feen and W.C. Welham. "The specific gravity of healthy men." *J.A.M.A.* 118(7): 495-498, 1942.

Beunen, G., M. Ostyn, R. Renson, J. Simons, D. Van Gerven. *Skeletal maturation and physical fitness of girls aged 12 through 16.* Hermes (Leuven), 445-457, 1976.

Borms, J., M. Hebbelinck, J.E.L. Carter, W.D. Ross, G. Larivière. Standardization of basic anthropometry in Olympic athletes — The MOGAP procedure. *Methods of Functional Anthropology.* U. Novotny and S. Titlbachova (eds). Charles University: Prague. 31-39, 1979.

Carter, J.E.L. Physical Structure of Olympic Athletes, Part 1. The Montreal Olympic Games Anthropological Project. J.E.L. Carter (ed). *Medicine and Sport.* p. 16, Karger: Basel, 16, 1982a.

Carter, J.E.L., W.D. Ross, S.P. Aubry, M. Hebbelinck, J. Borms. Anthropometry of Montreal Olympic Athletes. Physical structure of Olympic Athletes. Part 1. The Montreal Olympic Games Anthropological Project. J.E.L. Carter (ed). *Medicine and Sport,* 16, Karger: Basel, 25-52, 1982b.

Carter, J.E.L., S.P. Aubry, D.A. Sleet. Somatotypes of Montreal Olympic Athletes. Physical Structure of Olympic Athletes. Part 1. The Montreal Olympic Games Anthropological Project. J.E.L. Carter (ed). *Medicine and Sport,* 16, Karger: Basel, 53-80, 1981c.

Carter, J.E.L. *The Heath-Carter Somotype Method.* San Diego State University Syllabus Service, San Diego, 1980.

Carter, J.E.L. Somatotypes of female athletes. The Female Athlete. J. Borms and M. Hebbelinck (eds). *Medicine and Sport,* Karger, Basel, 85-116, 1981.

de Garay, A.L., L. Levine, J.E.L. Carter. *Genetic and Anthropological Studies of Olympic Athletes.* Academic Press: New York, 1977.

Drinkwater, D.T. and W.D. Ross. Anthropometric fractionation of body mass. *Kinanthropometry II.* M. Ostyn, G. Beunen, J. Simons (eds). Academic Press: Baltimore, 177-188, 1980.

Hirata, K. *Selection of Olympic Athletes,* Vol. 1 and 2, Hirata Institute of Health, 2234 Mino City, Gifu. Pref., Japan, 1977.

Leahy, R.M. A computer based error control and data monitoring system for anthropometric data (unpublished M.Sc. kinesiology thesis). Simon Fraser University, Burnaby, 1982.

Leahy, R.M., D.T. Drinkwater, G.R. Marshall, W.D. Ross. Computer solutions for longitudinal data: tri-dimensional computer graphics in the resolution of growth curves. *Kinanthropometry II.* M. Ostyn, G. Beunen, J. Simons. University Park Press: Baltimore, 425-441, 1980.

Malina, R.M., B.W. Meleski, R.F. Shoup. Anthropometric, body composition and maturity characteristics of selected school-age athletes. *Symposium in Sport.* Pediatric Clinics, North America, 29, 6, 1305-1323, 1982.

Malina, R.M., Menarche in Athletes: A synthesis and hypothesis. *Ann. Hum. Biol.,* 9, in press, 1982.

Marker, K. Influence of athletic training in the maturity process of girls. The Female Athlete. J. Borms, M. Hebbelinck, A. Venarando (eds). *Medicine and Sport,* 15, 117-126, Karger, Basel, 1981.

Martin, R. and K. Saller. *Lehrbuch der Anthropologie.* R. Gustav Fischer: Stuttgart, 1959.

Ross, W.D., S.R. Brown, R.A. Faulkner. Age of menarche in Canadian skaters and skiers. *Can. J. Ass. Sp. Sc.* 1: 163-167, 1977.

Ross, W.D., M.J. Marfell-Jones, D.R. Stirling, Prospects in Kinanthropometry. *The Sport Sciences,* J.T. Jackson and H.A. Wenger (eds). University of Victoria, Physical Education Series 4, 1982a.

Ross, W.D. and R. Ward. Sexual dimorphism and human proportionality. *Sexual Dimorphism in Homo Sapiens.* R. Hall (ed). Praeger: New York. 317-361, 1982b.

Ross, W.D., R.M. Leahy, D.T. Drinkwater, P.L. Swensen. Proportionality and body composition in male and female Olympic Athletes. *The Female Athlete.* J. Borms, M. Hebbelinck, A. Venerando (eds). 15, Karger: Basel 74-89, 1981.

Ross, W.D., D.T. Drinkwater, D.A. Bailey, G.R. Marshall, R.M. Leahy. Kinanthropometry: Traditions and new perspectives. *Kinanthropometry II,* M. Ostyn, G. Beunen, J. Simons (eds), University Park Press: Baltimore 372-378, 1980a.

Ross, W.D., D.T. Drinkwater, N.O. Whittingham and R.A. Faulkner. Anthropometric prototypes age 6 to 18 years. *Pediatric Work Physiology.* B.O. Ericsson and K. Berg (eds). Academic Press: Baltimore, 3-12, 1980b.

Ross, W.D. and R. Ward. Growth patterns, menarche and maturation in physically active girls. *The Female Athlete.* Proceedings of a National Conference about Women in Sport and Recreation. Simon Fraser University. A. Popma (ed). 63-71, 1980c.

Ross, W.D. and J.T. Corlett. Curriculum design in physical education; a scientific overview. *Promotion.* 4-10, 1980.

Ross, W.D., M. Hebbelinck, S.R. Brown, R.A. Faulkner. *Kinanthropometric landmarks and terminology.* R.J. Shepard and H. Lavallee (eds). Charles C. Thomas, Springfield, Ill., 44-50, 1978.

Ross, W.D., G.R. Marshall, A.S. Vajda, K. Roth. Dimensionalitat und Proportionalitat von Kraftleistungen. *Leisstungssport.* 8, 1, 195-205, 1978.

Ross, W.D., S.R. Brown, R.A. Faulkner, M.V. Savage. Monitoring growth in young skaters. *Can. J. Appl. Sp. Sc.,* 1: 163-167, 1977.

Siri, W.E. Body composition from fluid spaces and density: analysis of methods. *Technique for measuring body composition.* J. Brozek and A. Henschel (eds). National Academy of Science and National Research Council, Washington, D.C., 1961.

Siri, W.E. *Advances in Biological and Medical Physics.* Academic Press: New York. 1956.

Stewart, T.D. (ed.) *Hrdlicka's Practical Anthropometry.* The

Wistar Inst. of Anat. and Biol., Philadelphia, 1952.

Tanner, J.M., R.W. Whitehouse, W.A. Marshall, M.J.R. Healy. *Assessment of Skeletal Maturity and Prediction of Adult Stature.* (TW2 Method). Academic press, London, 1975.

Tanner, J.M. *Fetus Into Man.* Harvard University Press: Cambridge, Mass., 1978.

Weiner, J.S. and J.A. Lourie. *Practical Human Biology.* Academic Press: London, 1981.

APPENDIX 6.1

Table of Decimals of Year

In monitoring child growth, accurate records of the subject's date of birth and date of each measurement occasion are essential. Expressing age at any given time is awkward when months, weeks and days are used as units. The preferred procedure is to use decimal fractions of years to report a subject's age at any given measurement occasion. The table makes calculation easy. For example, if a girl was born on 6th April, 1963, and experienced her first menstrual flow on 15th August, 1975, the age of menarche would be determined as follows: 15 August, 1975 75.619; 6 April, 1963 63.260; Age of menarche 12.359.

	1 Jan.	2 Feb.	3 Mar.	4 Apr.	5 May	6 June	7 July	8 Aug.	9 Sept.	10 Oct.	11 Nov.	12 Dec.
1	000	085	162	247	329	414	496	581	666	748	833	915
2	003	088	164	249	332	416	499	584	668	751	836	918
3	005	090	167	252	334	419	501	586	671	753	838	921
4	008	093	170	255	337	422	504	589	674	756	841	923
5	011	096	173	258	340	425	507	592	677	759	844	926
6	014	099	175	260	342	427	510	595	679	762	847	929
7	015	101	178	263	345	430	512	597	682	764	849	932
8	019	104	181	266	348	433	515	600	685	767	852	934
9	022	107	184	268	351	436	518	603	688	770	855	937
10	025	110	186	271	353	438	521	605	690	773	858	940
11	027	112	189	274	356	441	523	608	693	775	860	942
12	030	115	192	277	359	444	526	611	696	778	863	945
13	033	118	195	279	362	447	529	614	699	781	866	948
14	036	121	197	282	364	449	532	616	701	784	868	951
15	038	123	200	285	367	452	534	619	704	786	871	953
16	041	126	203	288	370	455	537	622	707	789	874	956
17	044	129	205	290	373	458	540	625	710	792	877	959
18	047	132	208	293	375	460	542	627	712	795	879	962
19	049	134	211	296	378	463	545	630	715	797	882	964
20	052	137	214	299	381	466	548	633	718	800	885	967
21	055	140	216	301	384	468	551	636	721	803	888	970
22	058	142	219	304	386	471	553	638	723	805	890	973
23	060	145	222	307	389	474	556	641	726	808	893	975
24	063	148	225	310	392	477	559	644	729	811	896	978
25	066	151	227	312	395	479	562	647	731	814	899	981
26	068	153	230	315	397	482	564	649	734	816	901	984
27	071	156	233	318	400	485	567	652	737	819	904	986
28	074	159	236	321	403	488	570	655	740	822	907	989
29	077		238	323	405	490	573	658	742	825	910	992
30	079		241	326	408	493	575	660	745	827	912	995
31	082		244		411		578	663		830		997

| | Jan. 1 | Feb. 2 | Mar. 3 | Apr. 4 | May 5 | June 6 | July 7 | Aug. 8 | Sept. 9 | Oct. 10 | Nov. 11 | Dec. 12 |

APPENDIX 6.2

Factors to Convert Gas Volumes from Room Temperature, Saturated, to 37°C, Saturated

FACTOR TO CONVERT VOL. TO 37°C SAT.	WHEN GAS TEMPERATURE (°C)	WITH WATER VAPOR PRESSURE (MM HG) OF
1.102	20	17.5
1.096	21	18.7
1.091	22	19.8
1.085	23	21.1
1.080	24	22.4
1.075	25	23.8
1.068	26	25.2
1.063	27	26.7
1.057	28	28.3
1.051	29	30.0
1.045	30	31.8
1.039	31	33.7
1.032	32	35.7
1.026	33	37.7
1.020	34	39.9
1.014	35	42.2
1.007	36	44.6
1.000	37	47.0

The equation used is:

$$V_{(BTPS)} = \left(\frac{273 + 37}{273 + \text{room temp.}} \right) \times \left(\frac{\text{barometric pressure} - \begin{array}{c}\text{water vapor pressure corresponding}\\ \text{to gas temperature}\end{array}}{\text{barometric pressure} - 47} \right)$$

Water vapor pressure corresponding to gas at room temperature of 25°C is read from Table above.

Example:

$$V_{(BTPS)} = \left(\frac{273 + 37}{273 + 25} \right) \times \left(\frac{750 - 23.8}{750 - 47} \right) = 1.0746$$

APPENDIX 6.3

Descriptive Statistics for Canadian Reference Male and Female Students

VARIABLE	MALE STUDENTS (n = 153)			FEMALE STUDENTS (n = 94)		
	X̄	SD	range	X̄	SD	range
Age, years	21.3	2.85	17.6- 32.8	20.6	2.60	17.4- 30.6
Weight, kg	72.5	8.55	53.2-100.3	57.5	6.37	42.5- 76.4
Heights and lengths, cm						
Height	178.6	7.06	156.2-204.5	165.7	6.10	154.4-186.1
Sitting height	93.8	3.54	86.0-108.0	88.4	2.90	81.3- 94.7
Upper arm length	33.7	2.04	24.3- 39.9	31.1	1.76	27.8- 35.0
Forearm length	24.4	1.78	20.1- 36.5	22.7	1.44	19.8- 27.0
Upper extremity length	79.3	4.20	65.1-100.9	72.2	3.32	64.9- 81.9
Upper extremity — hand length	59.2	3.26	48.2- 72.1	53.8	2.86	48.1- 61.1
Ilio-spinal height	98.8	5.18	81.4-113.6	91.0	5.54	65.5-107.2
Lower extremity length	84.8	5.00	65.8- 96.9	77.3	4.26	69.8- 91.4
Thigh length	37.4	3.17	22.5- 44.1	34.6	2.24	30.7- 40.6
Tibial height	47.4	3.30	37.5- 69.9	42.7	2.34	37.4- 51.8
Foot length	26.5	1.36	22.8- 30.3	23.8	1.06	20.5- 26.4
Breadths, cm						
Biacromial breadth	40.0	2.05	34.3- 45.5	35.5	1.57	31.5- 39.6
Biiliocristal breadth	27.9	1.74	22.7- 37.5	27.5	1.87	23.1- 37.8
Transverse chest breadth	28.0	1.59	23.6- 32.2	24.5	1.34	21.2- 27.5
Anterior-posterior chest depth	19.6	1.58	15.9- 26.2	17.0	1.42	13.5- 20.1
Biepicondylar humerus breadth	7.2	0.37	6.3- 8.1	6.3	0.32	5.5- 7.2
Biepicondylar femur breadth	9.9	0.47	8.6- 11.1	8.9	0.43	7.9- 10.0
Girths, cm						
Arm girth (flexed and tensed)	32.4	2.40	24.7- 40.0	26.7	1.82	22.6- 32.8
Arm girth (relaxed)	30.0	2.34	23.1- 38.8	25.9	1.92	21.7- 31.6
Forearm girth (max. relaxed)	27.6	1.75	23.8- 34.0	23.6	1.50	20.2- 32.4
Wrist girth (prox. styloid)	17.0	0.83	14.9- 18.9	14.9	0.72	12.9- 17.6
Chest girth (mesosternal)	95.3	5.69	78.5-116.1	84.6	4.46	72.2- 98.8
Waist girth (minimum)	78.6	5.36	67.4- 96.9	68.0	4.17	58.8- 80.9
Thigh girth	55.9	4.43	47.2- 85.5	55.6	3.41	45.8- 64.7
Calf girth	37.1	2.19	32.5- 44.0	34.7	2.06	30.4- 39.9
Sum 6 skinfolds, mm	61.8	27.00	20.3-212.2	98.5	30.50	38.7-179.7

Data assembled in tri-university project by W.D. Ross (SFU), S.R.Brown (UBC), B. Howe (U. Victoria), to serve as CANREF control for Montreal Olympic Games Anthropological Project.
Carter et al. (1982a)

APPENDIX 6.4

Coquitlam Growth Study Age-Sex Prototypes

		G 06 n = 17	B 06 n = 15	G 07 n = 25	B 07 n = 22	G 08 n = 15	B 08 n = 22	G 09 n = 30	B 09 n = 27
Weight	Mean	21.38	21.75	23.52	23.92	25.12	27.50	28.74	28.80
	sd	3.69	2.98	3.94	2.85	3.81	4.53	5.02	5.15
Height		116.66	117.04	122.36	122.80	126.71	129.64	133.41	133.35
		5.68	6.30	5.25	5.07	4.99	6.01	6.56	7.37
Triceps sf		11.51	9.54	11.70	10.39	11.22	10.43	12.52	9.77
		3.24	2.01	4.37	2.18	2.68	3.43	3.37	3.21
Subscapular sf		7.14	6.02	7.41	6.28	5.86	6.94	7.14	6.88
		2.85	3.22	3.89	1.98	1.37	4.63	2.79	4.24
Suprailiac sf		5.23	4.76	6.28	4.93	5.51	6.32	6.46	5.74
		2.25	3.54	3.18	1.56	1.71	5.29	2.88	5.07
Abdominal sf		7.46	6.19	8.39	7.20	6.45	7.81	8.12	7.72
		2.63	5.58	5.19	2.50	2.01	5.70	3.12	6.38
Front thigh sf		17.87	12.88	16.88	15.22	15.97	15.25	18.71	15.20
		7.30	4.81	6.34	4.66	6.48	7.88	6.74	6.88
Medial calf sf		10.23	8.29	9.44	9.43	9.21	9.11	10.43	9.05
		3.41	1.97	3.73	2.77	3.89	3.88	3.02	4.12
Acromiale ht		90.64	90.86	95.20	96.18	99.58	102.49	105.38	104.80
		4.85	5.78	4.63	4.63	4.32	5.57	5.72	5.64
Radiale ht		69.51	70.19	73.40	74.15	76.67	78.87	81.04	80.91
		4.24	4.61	3.81	4.06	3.26	4.48	4.50	4.14
Stylion ht		53.32	53.84	56.55	56.86	59.21	60.43	62.49	62.32
		3.40	3.62	2.88	3.37	2.62	3.95	3.65	3.05
Dactylion ht		40.05	40.29	43.09	42.82	44.96	45.99	47.29	48.11
		2.79	2.64	2.60	3.00	2.17	3.55	3.26	2.87
Tibiale ht		28.74	29.20	31.08	30.96	32.95	33.27	34.95	34.71
		2.17	1.88	1.43	1.59	1.56	1.90	2.33	3.36
Spinale ht		60.84	61.36	64.98	64.96	68.59	69.43	72.94	71.79
		3.76	4.48	3.55	3.44	3.17	4.05	4.15	4.49
Gluteale ht		59.74	60.47	63.56	63.78	67.94	68.80	72.45	70.54
		4.05	4.12	4.32	3.65	3.17	4.04	4.19	4.47
Arm g (rel)		18.41	18.26	18.96	18.94	19.00	19.78	19.95	19.88
		1.95	2.49	2.22	1.14	1.72	2.22	1.91	2.15
Arm g (flex)		19.31	19.19	19.97	20.16	19.98	20.96	21.10	21.16
		1.91	2.66	2.31	1.23	1.43	2.09	2.10	2.07
Forearm girth		17.84	17.97	18.08	18.77	18.46	19.55	19.26	19.75
		1.47	1.41	1.39	0.91	1.15	1.41	1.40	1.42
Wrist girth		12.57	12.62	12.84	12.97	12.68	13.37	13.05	13.63
		0.94	0.79	1.24	0.78	0.77	0.96	0.90	1.42
Chest girth		58.92	58.90	60.86	61.40	62.47	64.06	64.73	66.20
		3.76	5.50	4.00	2.89	3.88	4.20	5.69	7.75
Waist girth		54.77	55.63	54.05	55.46	54.26	58.20	56.00	57.93
		4.11	4.96	4.87	2.66	2.78	3.95	4.68	4.06
Thigh girth		35.64	34.32	38.22	36.45	37.28	38.37	40.71	39.26
		3.67	5.24	3.99	2.51	4.45	3.79	4.32	3.94
Calf girth		24.28	24.03	24.75	25.15	25.32	26.32	26.59	27.18
		2.01	1.79	1.98	1.63	1.75	1.90	2.17	3.10
Ankle girth		16.71	16.30	16.88	17.08	16.96	17.76	17.98	18.17
		1.33	1.36	1.21	1.01	1.20	1.15	1.32	1.47
Bi-acromial br		24.96	25.59	26.13	26.65	27.63	28.17	28.98	28.63
		1.42	1.37	1.68	1.19	1.77	1.29	1.69	1.91
Bi-iliocr br		18.47	18.68	19.58	19.56	19.76	20.54	20.67	20.46
		1.23	0.88	2.50	1.95	1.49	1.93	1.30	1.44

Trans chest	17.27	18.10	18.36	18.52	18.50	19.25	19.17	19.42
	1.04	0.89	2.28	1.04	1.13	1.50	1.22	1.22
Foot length	17.56	17.63	18.41	18.57	19.19	19.56	20.29	20.13
	1.08	1.20	1.00	1.26	1.36	1.12	1.08	1.32
Bi-epi hum wd	4.94	5.10	4.98	5.24	5.09	5.50	5.37	5.57
	0.40	0.51	0.30	0.26	0.30	0.34	0.30	0.36
Bi-epi fem wd	7.13	7.47	7.38	7.70	7.44	8.05	7.76	8.13
	0.46	0.44	0.38	0.39	0.42	0.37	0.50	0.77
Sitting ht	64.99	65.18	66.83	67.48	68.35	69.99	71.29	71.54
	3.19	3.00	2.33	2.71	3.09	2.92	3.35	3.20
A-P chest	12.87	13.47	12.93	13.54	13.44	14.06	13.32	14.31
	1.24	0.74	0.88	0.93	1.00	1.01	0.96	1.10
Head girth	51.11	51.80	51.16	52.45	51.61	53.03	52.30	52.54
	1.66	0.93	1.77	1.76	1.17	1.18	1.15	1.10
Neck girth	25.66	26.83	26.06	27.16	26.49	28.24	26.88	27.99
	1.64	1.31	1.33	1.93	1.06	1.74	1.39	1.63

COGRO Prototypes (continued)

	G 10 n = 20	B 10 n = 21	G 11 n = 24	B 11 n = 26	G 12 n = 35	B 12 n = 33	G 13 n = 37	B 13 n = 35
Weight	35.84	33.23	39.12	37.21	42.79	42.18	47.92	48.00
	9.18	5.90	10.22	7.95	7.95	8.61	9.44	7.46
Height	141.52	140.14	145.15	143.15	152.89	149.25	159.33	159.20
	8.19	6.99	7.78	6.89	7.84	6.45	7.00	6.94
Triceps sf	13.16	9.94	14.28	10.03	13.43	13.15	13.04	11.58
	5.41	3.64	4.18	3.39	4.62	7.20	4.85	6.16
Subscapular sf	11.09	7.11	10.20	7.95	9.97	11.16	11.09	8.70
	8.13	3.75	4.50	5.72	3.66	8.52	6.75	5.83
Suprailiac sf	9.65	5.79	10.00	6.74	10.57	11.21	11.12	8.46
	6.20	3.45	5.45	4.83	5.23	8.60	6.25	9.35
Abdominal sf	12.31	8.81	13.14	9.85	13.19	14.60	14.61	12.38
	8.63	7.40	6.46	8.83	6.75	1.73	7.86	9.38
Front thigh sf	22.60	17.67	23.53	16.99	23.65	21.53	21.45	16.45
	10.23	7.86	8.16	5.32	9.15	2.33	7.79	7.64
Medial calf sf	12.97	9.70	12.90	10.01	14.18	13.50	13.25	11.18
	6.65	4.41	5.45	3.59	4.81	8.52	4.76	5.57
Acromiale ht	113.61	110.90	116.07	115.60	123.58	119.92	128.31	127.84
	8.41	6.76	6.84	6.28	6.40	5.47	5.91	6.01
Radiale ht	88.02	86.40	89.00	88.93	95.27	92.40	98.64	98.24
	7.14	5.24	5.44	4.98	5.44	4.50	4.75	4.99
Stylion ht	67.98	66.10	68.38	68.26	73.30	70.69	75.79	75.00
	5.55	4.64	4.48	4.05	4.71	3.60	3.69	6.87
Dactylion ht	52.62	50.86	53.12	52.55	57.10	54.76	58.71	57.56
	4.66	3.80	3.83	3.40	3.75	3.18	3.28	3.16
Tibiale ht	37.57	36.87	37.97	38.30	40.87	39.02	42.39	43.06
	3.08	2.58	2.46	2.66	2.41	2.51	2.23	2.57
Spinale ht	79.46	77.33	80.77	80.30	86.01	83.29	89.59	89.77
	6.14	5.33	4.80	4.89	4.47	4.42	4.67	4.22
Gluteale ht	77.10	75.56	77.99	77.68	83.85	81.36	88.05	87.41
	5.45	4.92	5.18	5.16	4.46	4.92	4.54	4.73
Arm g (rel)	22.11	20.88	22.27	21.32	23.09	32.66	23.58	24.13
	3.14	2.46	2.58	2.28	2.76	3.52	2.83	2.37
Arm g (flex)	23.32	22.43	23.59	22.84	24.19	25.19	24.56	26.03
	2.88	2.29	2.68	2.18	2.55	3.39	2.73	2.59
Forearm girth	20.79	20.61	21.00	21.25	21.77	22.50	22.32	23.55
	1.89	1.36	1.75	1.45	1.78	2.00	1.65	1.54

Wrist girth	13.81	14.03	14.12	14.10	14.70	14.87	14.82	15.55
	1.15	1.08	1.03	1.04	1.20	1.37	1.10	0.91
Chest girth	70.38	69.69	71.45	70.83	74.22	74.23	78.73	79.55
	6.90	5.18	6.05	6.15	5.76	6.77	6.17	5.98
Waist girth	59.51	61.31	61.17	62.01	62.13	66.03	64.41	68.11
	6.56	5.32	5.79	5.65	5.32	7.70	6.05	5.57
Thigh girth	45.50	41.55	45.89	42.71	48.25	46.50	49.31	48.20
	6.15	3.90	5.24	2.95	5.44	5.74	5.68	4.47
Calf girth	28.58	27.77	29.55	29.11	30.80	30.91	32.14	32.36
	3.19	1.92	3.14	2.34	2.51	3.24	2.97	2.50
Ankle girth	19.30	18.93	19.85	19.43	20.21	20.43	21.00	21.20
	2.28	1.34	1.95	1.48	1.72	2.20	1.45	1.61
Bi-acromial br	30.73	30.40	30.50	31.01	32.00	31.79	33.88	34.29
	1.51	1.43	2.53	1.95	2.39	3.16	2.11	1.91
Bi-iliocr br	22.32	21.72	23.12	22.42	24.06	23.19	25.29	24.95
	2.12	1.58	2.53	1.40	2.52	1.80	2.48	3.47
Trans chest	20.62	20.96	20.73	21.09	21.63	21.77	22.96	23.45
	1.64	1.56	1.65	1.73	2.03	1.58	2.18	1.48
Foot length	21.26	21.52	21.75	22.21	22.71	22.92	23.42	24.46
	1.62	2.19	1.43	1.41	1.24	1.07	1.29	1.47
Bi-epi hum wd	5.64	5.93	5.75	6.06	6.02	6.25	6.21	6.54
	0.37	0.39	0.42	0.77	0.45	0.67	0.42	0.68
Bi-epi fem wd	8.29	8.52	8.46	8.66	8.74	8.99	8.76	9.54
	0.70	0.52	0.53	0.51	0.52	0.52	0.51	0.48
Sitting ht	75.13	74.09	76.22	75.27	79.41	77.77	82.86	81.82
	4.00	3.93	4.28	2.99	4.15	3.04	4.16	4.06
A-P chest	15.14	14.58	15.30	15.28	15.48	16.17	16.32	17.12
	1.70	0.95	1.56	1.44	1.21	1.52	1.34	1.49
Head girth	52.81	54.02	53.02	53.45	53.24	53.55	53.82	54.59
	1.42	1.53	1.50	1.18	1.92	1.51	1.54	1.24
Neck girth	28.20	28.94	28.79	29.46	29.37	30.08	30.40	31.91
	2.12	1.31	2.08	1.93	1.84	1.12	1.91	1.70

COGRO Prototypes (continued)

	G 14 n = 67	B 14 n = 76	G 15 n = 66	B 15 n = 77	G 16 n = 53	B 16 n = 55	G 17 n = 47	B 17 n = 43	G 18 n = 10	B 18 n = 21
Weight	52.42	52.60	53.89	58.63	54.87	62.16	55.76	64.86	59.51	68.82
	9.44	9.69	7.57	11.23	8.03	8.86	6.79	9.85	6.44	7.70
Height	162.53	165.52	163.12	170.46	164.61	174.59	165.13	175.63	165.88	179.04
	6.19	8.64	6.77	8.73	6.64	8.37	5.69	6.23	7.23	7.66
Triceps sf	14.57	9.96	15.05	9.64	14.48	8.93	16.15	9.46	17.01	9.40
	4.84	4.35	4.68	4.62	4.38	3.75	4.56	5.18	3.73	2.62
Subscapular sf	11.72	8.28	11.95	9.46	11.72	8.63	11.10	8.92	12.61	8.79
	5.74	4.43	5.47	6.83	5.51	4.21	4.22	4.72	3.82	1.56
Suprailiac sf	12.26	7.76	11.70	8.43	11.83	8.25	11.08	7.36	11.71	6.25
	5.89	4.84	5.18	6.39	5.34	5.55	3.98	5.29	4.43	1.67
Abdominal sf	16.83	10.89	16.16	11.63	16.42	11.47	14.91	10.87	15.84	10.47
	8.14	7.16	6.94	8.70	8.31	8.75	5.51	6.96	4.41	3.67
Front thigh sf	23.21	14.63	24.74	14.50	24.16	13.10	25.66	12.13	24.85	12.66
	7.65	6.33	7.31	7.61	7.14	7.26	7.35	5.70	6.63	4.16
Medial calf sf	14.79	10.45	15.21	10.36	15.02	9.96	16.33	9.48	15.44	9.08
	5.64	4.62	5.26	5.26	5.88	5.46	5.44	4.98	3.03	3.33
Acromiale ht	130.46	132.77	131.12	137.14	132.64	140.63	133.06	140.91	133.37	143.49
	5.43	7.15	6.26	7.19	5.93	7.50	5.78	5.38	7.05	7.57
Radiale ht	100.43	101.99	101.00	105.47	102.10	107.90	102.38	107.78	102.64	109.45
	4.19	5.46	4.69	5.74	4.36	6.11	4.78	4.44	5.94	6.43
Stylion ht	77.32	78.18	78.1	80.83	78.74	82.39	78.55	81.99	78.62	83.32
	3.46	4.33	3.80	4.81	3.49	4.94	4.08	3.68	5.18	5.15

Dactylion ht	60.10	60.17	60.67	62.45	61.19	63.86	61.35	63.04	61.08	64.39
	2.98	3.41	3.59	4.04	3.05	4.46	3.53	3.46	4.14	4.66
Tibiale ht	42.55	44.42	42.31	45.49	42.94	45.84	42.51	45.36	42.44	46.41
	1.99	2.89	2.22	2.91	2.01	2.32	2.64	2.33	3.59	3.17
Spinale ht	89.97	92.76	89.57	95.35	90.87	97.19	90.96	96.90	91.59	98.58
	4.24	5.43	6.17	5.62	4.56	5.03	4.59	4.16	5.79	5.69
Gluteale ht	88.53	90.64	88.51	92.75	88.73	93.73	88.41	92.53	88.74	94.31
	4.22	5.25	4.51	5.63	3.88	4.88	5.11	4.36	1.36	5.92
Arm g (rel)	24.99	24.75	25.53	26.27	25.36	27.28	26.07	28.57	27.57	29.18
	2.83	2.52	2.37	2.95	2.42	2.17	2.16	3.21	1.85	1.92
Arm g (flex)	26.35	26.79	26.71	28.72	26.62	29.83	27.27	31.25	28.66	31.58
	2.76	2.66	2.22	3.28	2.46	2.35	2.04	2.98	1.82	2.01
Forearm girth	23.30	24.48	23.52	25.56	23.59	26.38	23.96	26.87	24.37	27.31
	1.55	1.81	1.86	2.00	1.31	2.07	1.45	1.63	1.16	1.16
Wrist girth	15.47	16.04	15.38	16.49	15.44	16.86	15.38	16.95	15.32	17.46
	1.20	1.23	1.15	1.21	0.78	0.92	0.69	1.05	0.53	0.71
Chest girth	81.94	82.03	82.26	86.25	82.74	87.97	82.45	90.25	84.84	93.03
	5.40	6.41	4.87	7.80	5.28	5.60	3.82	6.56	3.77	3.68
Waist girth	66.56	68.31	65.15	70.76	66.10	72.28	66.21	74.68	67.23	75.64
	5.97	5.72	4.84	6.60	6.29	5.40	3.94	7.72	2.52	3.78
Thigh girth	52.75	49.12	53.69	51.46	53.91	52.80	55.23	53.82	57.04	55.30
	5.26	5.14	3.79	5.68	4.89	4.50	4.29	5.16	3.62	3.54
Calf girth	33.60	33.29	34.23	34.46	34.34	35.35	34.62	35.91	26.32	36.70
	2.76	3.01	2.53	2.82	2.56	2.48	2.41	2.98	2.05	2.33
Ankle girth	21.55	21.74	21.45	22.35	21.43	22.71	21.18	22.36	21.53	22.94
	1.58	1.62	1.26	1.68	1.35	1.31	1.25	1.52	1.33	1.25
Bi-acromial br	34.95	35.55	34.93	36.86	35.35	37.56	35.30	38.26	34.65	39.27
	1.84	2.36	2.06	2.38	2.49	3.03	1.76	2.58	2.55	2.16
Bi-iliocr br	26.20	25.01	26.34	26.01	26.57	26.67	27.10	27.35	27.82	27.44
	1.96	1.85	2.02	1.81	1.46	1.82	1.82	1.94	1.21	1.39
Trans chest	32.50	24.21	23.57	25.41	24.42	26.57	24.66	27.21	25.43	27.80
	1.85	1.44	2.02	2.11	1.49	1.80	1.82	1.92	1.68	1.50
Foot length	23.57	25.27	23.38	25.46	23.37	25.79	23.40	25.79	23.81	26.41
	1.13	1.51	1.08	1.41	1.01	1.47	1.29	1.03	1.08	1.27
Bi-epi hum wd	6.31	6.89	6.25	7.09	6.29	7.13	6.17	7.05	6.26	7.24
	0.34	0.47	0.36	0.47	0.26	0.40	0.33	0.36	0.32	0.37
Bi-epi fem wd	8.93	9.61	8.82	9.74	8.87	9.79	9.02	9.71	8.94	9.93
	0.47	0.58	0.56	0.56	0.44	0.49	0.47	0.52	0.39	0.50
Sitting ht	85.16	85.08	86.23	87.78	86.94	90.69	87.54	91.76	87.98	93.09
	3.45	4.38	3.25	5.24	3.19	5.16	4.56	3.44	1.80	3.06
A-P chest	16.67	17.46	16.75	18.16	16.66	18.23	16.67	18.70	17.62	18.97
	1.59	1.68	1.70	1.89	1.53	1.72	1.34	1.36	0.77	1.22
Head girth	53.33	55.28	54.07	55.77	54.10	56.16	53.73	55.68	54.37	56.70
	1.35	1.74	1.44	1.61	1.32	1.44	1.56	1.75	1.92	1.85
Neck girth	31.06	32.81	31.22	34.07	30.90	34.84	30.67	35.41	31.53	36.79
	1.50	2.42	1.75	2.75	1.72	1.82	1.26	2.13	1.12	1.76

APPENDIX 6.5

Phantom Specifications

	p	s
Stature (stretch) cm	170.18	6.29
Body mass, weight kg	64.58	8.60
Lean body mass kg	52.45	6.14
Fat mass kg	12.13	3.25
Percent fat	18.78	5.20
Density g·cm^{-3}	1.056	0.011
Bone mass kg	10.49	1.57
Muscle mass kg	25.55	2.99
Residual body mass kg	16.41	1.90
H in/$\sqrt[3]{W}$ lb	12.83	
H cm/$\sqrt[3]{W}$ kg	42.41	
($\sqrt[3]{W}$ kg/H cm) × 10^3	23.58	
Somatotype*	5·4·2½	

*Heath and Carter (1976).

Phantom Heights (Projected)

	p	s
Vertex (stretch stature)	170.18	6.29
Gnathion	148.81	5.65
Suprasternal	138.31	5.46
Infrasternal	119.50	4.96
Symphysion	87.05	4.35
Acromial	139.37	5.45
Radial	107.25	5.36
Stylion	82.68	4.13
Dactylion	63.83	3.38
Iliospinal*	94.11	4.71
Trochanteric*	86.40	4.32
Tibial (lateral or medial)*	44.82	2.56
Sphyrion (fibular)	7.10	0.85
Sphyrion (tibial)	8.01	0.96
Cervical	144.15	5.58
Gluteal arch*	88.33	4.41
Sitting height*	89.92	4.50
Span (dactylion-dactylion)	172.35	7.41

*These data revised from Ross and Wilson (1976).

Phantom Lengths (Derived and Direct)

	p	s
Head height (vertex-gnathion)	27.27	1.02
Neck (gnathion-suprasternale)	9.48	1.71
Trunk (suprasternale-symphysion)	51.26	2.56
Back (cervicale-gluteal arch)	56.83	2.84
Upper extremity (acromiale-dactylion)	75.95	3.64
Upper extremity (acromiale-stylion)	57.10	2.74
Arm (acromiale-radiale)	32.53	1.77
Forearm (radiale-stylion)	24.57	1.37
Hand (stylion-dactylion)	18.85	0.85
Lower extremity length (stature-sitting height)*	81.06	4.05
Thigh 1 (stature-sitting height-tibiale)*	35.44	2.12
Thigh 2 (iliospinale-tibiale)*	49.29	2.96
Thigh 3 (trochanterion-tibiale)*	41.37	2.48
Tibia (tibiale mediale-t. sphyrion)*	36.81	2.10
Lower leg (tibiale laterale-f. sphyrion)*	37.72	2.15
Foot length (standing, akropodion-pternion)*	25.50	1.16
Foot length (flat unweighted, akropodion-pternion)*	24.81	1.15

*These data revised from Ross and Wilson (1976).

Phantom Girths

	p	s
Head	56.00	1.44
Neck	34.91	1.73
Shoulders	104.86	6.23
Chest (mesosternale, end tidal)	87.86	5.18
Abdominal 1 (waist)	71.91	4.45
Abdominal 2 (umbilical)	79.06	6.95
Abdominal AV (mean 1 and 2)	75.48	5.74
Hips	94.67	5.58
Thigh (1 cm distal, gluteal line)	55.82	4.23
Knee	36.04	2.17
Calf (standing)	35.25	2.30
Ankle	21.71	1.33
Arm (fully flexed and tensed)	29.41	2.37
Arm (relaxed, mid-acromiale-radiale)	26.89	2.33
Forearm (relaxed)	25.13	1.41
Wrist 1 (distal styloids)	16.35	0.72
Wrist 2 (proximal styloids)	16.38	0.72
Arm girth relaxed ($-\pi$ × triceps skinfold cm)*	22.05	1.91
Chest girth ($-\pi$ × subscapular skinfold cm)*	82.46	4.86
Thigh girth ($-\pi$ × front thigh skinfold cm)*	47.34	3.59
Calf girth ($-\pi$ × medial calf skinfold cm)*	30.22	1.97

*Fat-corrected girths for fractionation of body mass procedure.

Phantom Breadths

	p	s
Biacromial	38.04	1.92
Bideltoid	43.50	2.40
Transverse chest (mesosternale)	27.92	1.74
Biiliocristal	28.84	1.75
Bitrochanteric	32.66	1.80
Chest depth (AP, mesosternale)	17.50	1.38
Biepicondylar humerus	6.48	0.35
Wrist (max. stylion-ulnare)	5.21	0.28
Hand (distal II-V metacarpals)	8.28	0.50
Biepicondylar femur	9.52	0.48
Transverse tibia	9.12	0.47
Bimalleolare	6.68	0.36
Transverse foot (standing)	9.61	0.60
Transverse foot (resting flat unweighted)	8.96	0.56
Foot (standing, distal I-V metatarsals)	10.34	0.65

Phantom Skinfolds (Harpenden Caliper)

	p	s
Triceps	15.4	4.47
Subscapular (diagonal)	17.2	5.07
Subscapular (vertical)	17.5	5.17
Chest	11.8	3.27
Biceps	8.0	2.00
Suprailiac	15.4	4.47
Abdominal	25.4	7.78
Iliac crest	22.4	6.80
Front thigh	27.0	8.33
Rear thigh	31.1	9.69
Medial calf	16.0	4.67

Phantom Head and Face Measures

	p	s
Classic head height (vertex-gnathion)	27.27	1.02
Head length (glabella-occiput)	19.15	0.68
Head breadth (transverse parietal)	15.08	0.58
Head height (vertex-tragion)	13.31	0.75
Bizygomatic breadth	13.66	0.57
Bigonial breadth	10.59	0.58
Morphological face height (nasion-gnathion)	11.94	0.69
Nose length (nasion-subnasale)	5.21	0.48

APPENDIX 6.6

Anthropometric Measurement Tolerances

Body Weight	.5 kg
Height	3 mm
Acromial Height	2 mm
Radial Height	2 mm
Stylion Height	2 mm
Dactylion Height	2 mm
Trochanter Height	2 mm
Spinal Height	2 mm
Malleolar Height	2 mm
Sitting Height	2 mm
Tibial Height	1-2 mm
Bicondylar Humerus Width	1 mm
Bicondylar Femur Width	1 mm
Biacromial Diameter	1-2 mm
Thorax Diameter Transv.	2-3 mm
Thorax Diameter Sagit.	1-2 mm
Bi-iliocristal Diameter	1-2 mm
Wrist Width	1-2 mm
Neck Girth	2 mm
Upper Arm Extended	2 mm
Upper Arm Flexed	2 mm
Chest Girth Inspiration	1-2%
† Chest Girth Expiration	1-2%
Waist Girth	2-3%
Abdomen Girth	1 mm
Thigh Girth	1 mm
Calf Girth	1 mm
† Skinfolds	5%
* Forearm Girth	2 mm
* Wrist Girth	1 mm
* Ankle Girth	1 mm
* Foot Girth	1 mm
* Head Girth	1 mm

Adapted from Borms et al. (1979).

†Percentage of the sample mean was used.
*Included by Leahy (1982).

Testing Flexibility

Cheryl Hubley

INTRODUCTION

Flexibility is defined as the range of motion at a single joint or a series of joints. Attempts have been made to differentiate static and dynamic flexibility. A rigorous definition of the latter term, however, has not been universally accepted. Thus, many authors refer to flexibility as a static measure.

It should be noted that flexibility does not exist as a general characteristic but is specific to the joint and joint action (Hupprich and Sigerseth, 1950; Harris, 1969, and Munroe and Romance, 1975). This is an important factor to consider when designing a test battery for athletes involved in different sports.

A review of the literature indicates that flexibility is of interest to coaches, physical educators, sports scientists, and rehabilitation therapists. Generally they agree that it is an important element of athletic performance, injury prevention, and rehabilitation. Based on such a large interest group, one would expect an abundance of well documented information on measuring procedures and training techniques. This is not the case, and it is the hope of this author that the following presentation will stimulate members of these groups to conduct research to improve, develop, and validate flexibility measuring procedures. Since sport involves both statics and dynamics, research efforts should focus on the development of measuring techniques for both.

Limiting Factors

Several factors limit the range of motion at a joint. The structure of the joint and the interface between the two articulating surfaces can prevent excessive ranges of motion at different joints. For example, the ulnar-humeral articulation is a freely moveable hinge joint, but movement is restricted to flexion and extension in the sagittal plane. A summary of the classification and movements permitted at some major joints of the body is found in Table 7.1.

The soft tissues surrounding the joint, such as

Table 7.1 Classification and movements permitted by some major joints of the body

CLASSIFICATION	JOINTS	MOVEMENT
Ball and socket	Hip Shoulder	Flexion/extension Abduction/adduction Internal/external rotation
Hinge	Ankle Elbow	Flexion/extension
Modified hinge	Knee	Flexion/extension Some rotation
Pivot	Radial-ulnar	Supination/pronation
Gliding	Spinal column	Flexion/extension Lateral flexion Spinal rotation

muscles, tendons, fascia, ligaments, and skin, also restrict joint motion (Johns and Wright, 1962). Certain pathologies or injuries also may limit the range of motion at the affected joint (Klafs and Arnheim, 1973).

It is obvious that the boney structures and articular cartilage of the joint should not be altered. Therefore, the soft tissues surrounding the joint must be stretched to increase range of motion.

Factors Affecting Flexibility

Several variables have been proposed as possible factors affecting flexibility measurements. Some of the variables examined include age, sex, body type, and exercise. These studies do not provide conclusive evidence that any of these factors has an effect on flexibility. The discrepancies presented in these studies lead to the general conclusion that the habitual movement patterns of the individual are more important, with sex and age being secondary considerations.

Preliminary evidence shows that warm-up and external temperature do affect range of motion measures (Fieldman, 1967; Cotton and Waters, 1970; Grobaker and Stull, 1975). These studies do not establish the magnitude of the influence but provide an initial indication that both warm-up and environmental temperature should be controlled during flexibility testing.

Trainability

There are three basic techniques used to increase flexibility: *static stretching, ballistic stretching*, and *Proprioceptive Neuromuscular Facilitation* (PNF). The ballistic method relies on bouncing and momentum to stretch the soft tissues surrounding the joint. This method generally is not advocated because of the possibility of injury to these structures. Static stretching is merely assuming a stretched position and holding that position for a period of time. There is little chance of injury using this method. Studies comparing the increases in flexibility between the static and the ballistic stretching techniques showed no significant differences (Logan and Egstrom, 1961; deVries, 1962, and Holt et al., 1970).

The PNF technique utilizes an isometric contraction of the muscle to be stretched, followed by relaxation of that muscle and contraction of the antagonist. Studies have shown that the PNF method is superior for increasing range of motion

compared to other techniques (Holt et al., 1970; Tanigawa, 1972, and Moore and Hutton, 1980).

Although norms have been published for non-athletic male subjects (Boone and Azen, 1979) there are presently no normative values of acceptable ranges of motion or increases in range of motion for athletes. Individuals must realize their limit and perceive excessive pain or discomfort as the body's injury prevention mechanism.

The effects due to any of the stretching techniques are lost shortly after the exercises are completed (Tanigawa, 1972). Therefore, daily stretching routines should become a part of the athlete's training program.

PURPOSE OF TESTING FLEXIBILITY

It has been suggested that flexibility is an important component of sports performance, injury prevention, and rehabilitation. As early as 1941, Cureton proposed that flexibility was an integral part of physical fitness. A few individuals have correlated selected flexibility measures with performance measures but were unable to determine a true causal relationship between these variables (Leighton, 1957; Burley et al., 1961, and Dentiman, 1964). Based on the present literature, there is no scientific evidence linking flexibility to performance. An analysis of numerous athletic performances, however, clearly shows that extreme ranges of motion are assumed in many activities. Some examples are provided in Figure 7.1.

Stretching and increasing range of motion have been considered an effective method of preventing injuries to the muscles, ligaments, and tendons of the body (Klafs and Arnheim, 1973; Austin, 1977; Kresci and Koch, 1979, and Kuland et al., 1979). Several researchers have concluded that mobilization and loading, if not too excessive, do increase the strength of the bone and ligament or tendon complex (Rigby et al., 1958; Rasch et al., 1960; Laros et al., 1971; Noyes et al., 1974; Tipton et al., 1975, and Weisman et al., 1980). No evidence is available, however, which proves that flexibility actually reduces the number or severity of injuries to athletes. On the other hand, it has been shown quite clearly that the structures injured most frequently in sports are the muscles, tendons, and ligaments (Kennedy and Hawkins, 1974; Kalemak and Morehouse, 1975; Kennedy et al., 1978; Berson et al., 1978; Kuland et al., 1979; Johnson et al., 1979; Glick, 1980; Renstrom and Peterson, 1980, and Smodlaka, 1980).

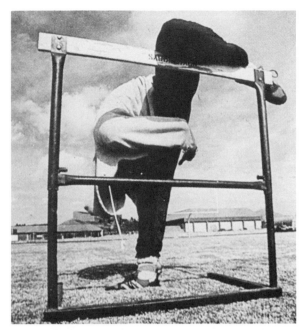

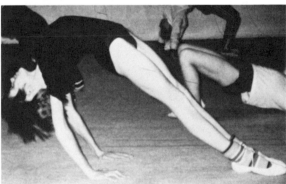

Fig. 7.1 Examples of extreme range of motion.

Often, exercises prescribed as part of the rehabilitative program are performed through the full range of motion possible at the injured joint (Knight, 1979, and Smodlaka, 1980). Such procedures indicate the importance of restoring the full range of motion as a necessary element of the rehabilitation process.

In conclusion, the evidence presented is mostly speculative with few sound scientific studies backing the claim that flexibility is important to sport. The basic concept that flexibility is a necessity for athletes, however, is shared by individuals from several disciplines. Therefore, the purpose for measuring range of motion is to have a quantita-tive value that can be compared within and between individuals. These measures could be used to assess improvements and to identify problem areas associated with poor performance or possible injury.

RELEVANCE

The relevance of flexibility to sport can be reflected best simply by observing skills and movement patterns associated with different sports. It would be a tedious task to list all the movement patterns and to identify all the joints where full or extreme ranges of motion are required. Therefore, as a coach of a sport, one must develop the ability to evaluate skills and identify the joints and joint actions pertinent to successful completion of the skills. Table 7.2 lists a few sports and indicates the joints where mobility is required to perform the skills associated with that sport. This table is by no means all-inclusive but it does provide a general guide.

TESTING PROCEDURES

Several testing procedures for measuring flexibility are described in the literature. These are generally divided into direct and indirect techniques.

Indirect Methods

The indirect methods usually involve linear measures of distances between segments or from an external object. The most popular techniques described are the standing and sitting toe touch tests (Cureton, 1941; Kraus and Hirshland, 1954; Wells and Dillan, 1952, and Fleishman, 1963). Three of these techniques are presented as examples.

Cureton's Test for Minimal Level of Flexibility

1. Floor touch. Subject stands with hands by side, then leans forward slowly and touches floor with fingertips while keeping knees straight.

To pass, men touch fingertips to floor, and women touch palms to floor.

2. Trunk forward bend. Subject sits on a table, legs straight, and bends forward as far as possible.

The distance from the forehead to the table is measured.

Table 7.2   Joint actions associated with performance of skills in some major sports

SPORT	HIP	KNEE	ANKLE	SHOULDER	ELBOW	WRIST	TRUNK
Hurdles	Add/Abd Fl/Ex IR/ER	Fl/Ex					
High Jump	Fl/Ex	Fl/Ex					
Diving	Fl/Ex	Fl/Ex	Fl/Ex	Fl/Ex			Fl/Ex Rot
Swimming	Fl/Ex Add/Abd IR/ER		Fl/Ex In/Ev	Fl/Ex Add/Abd IR/ER			
Pitching	Fl/Ex			Fl/Ex Add/Abd IR/ER	S/P Fl/Ex	Fl/Ex	Rot
Soccer	Fl/Ex IR/ER Add/Abd	Fl/Ex	Fl/Ex In/Ev				
Speed Skating	Add/Abd Fl/Ex IR/ER	Fl/Ex	Fl/Ex				
Gymnastics	Fl/Ex Add/Abd IR/ER	Fl/Ex	Fl/Ex	Fl/Ex Add/Abd IR/ER	Fl/Ex	Fl/Ex	Fl/Ex Rot

S — supination	Add — adduction
P — pronation	Abd — abduction
In — inversion	Fl — flexion
Ev — eversion	Ex — extension
Rot — rotation	IR — internal rotation
	ER — external rotation

3. Trunk extension. Subject lies in prone position on a table with feet secured, then raises head and chest.

The distance from the forehead to the table is measured.

Kraus-Weber Floor Touch Test

Test was designed to measure length of back and hamstring muscles. Subject stands in bare or stocking feet, hands by sides, feet together, knees straight, then leans forward slowly to touch floor and holds for three seconds with no bouncing.

Pass or fail.

Wells and Dillan Test

The following tests were compared as methods of measuring leg and back flexibility.

1. Standing bobbing. Subject stands on gymnasium bench letting arms and trunk relax forward.

Subject bobs four times then holds position of maximum stretch.

Measures are taken from bench to fingertips; above bench are negative, below are positive.

2. Sit and reach. Subject sits on floor with legs straddling a bar bench. Subject bobs forward four times and holds maximum position. Measurements are taken from fingertips to a zero mark on the floor.

These tests do not provide an accurate measure of joint range of motion, as values are affected by the anthropometrics of the individual (Broer and Galles, 1958, and Wear, 1963). Therefore, indirect tests do not provide adequate information for our purposes but can be useful for within-subject comparisons.

Direct Methods

The goniometer (see Figure 7.2) often is used to measure range of motion at a joint in degrees. The center of the goniometer is positioned at the axis of rotation of the joint, and the arms of the goniometer are aligned with the long axis of the bones of adjacent segments. The goniometer recently has been criticized and no longer is considered a reliable tool for measuring range of motion (Markas, 1979; Speakman and Kung, 1978). The two major problems with this measuring device are identifying the axis of motion for complex actions (Moore, 1979) and positioning the arms of the goniometer along the bones of the segments (Harris, 1969).

The Leighton flexometer (1942) (see Figure 7.3) is another instrument designed to measure directly range of motion. The flexometer consists of a gravity needle and a strap attachment for the limb. The flexometer can be used to measure range of motion at several joints and for different joint actions. These actions are listed in Figure 7.4. The reliability coefficients reported in the literature for this device all are very good (Hupprich and Sigerseth, 1950; Sigerseth and Haluski, 1950; Mathews et al., 1957; Harris, 1969, and Munroe and Romance, 1975). The major problem cited in the literature is that the flexometer does not distinguish adequately between hip and back range of motion (Twomey and Taylor, 1979).

Radiography has been considered by some individuals to be the most valid means of measuring range of motion (Kott and Mundale, 1959). Although this may be true especially for some movements, there are obvious problems associated with radioactive exposure, accessibility of equipment, and training of personnel.

Finally, there is the electrogoniometer, which measures joint angles during activity (Karpovich and Karpovich, 1959). It is conceivable that, with more research and development, this instrument could be used to measure dynamic ranges of motion.

RECOMMENDED TESTING PROCEDURES

There is no technique presently available which measures the composite range of motion at several joints during a specific sport movement. The best alternative, based on the present literature, is the Leighton flexometer. There are six basic reasons for this conclusion:

1. It gives a direct quantification of range of motion in degrees.
2. The starting position is standardized due to the gravity needle.
3. The investigator does not have to locate or assume a joint center of rotation; placement of the flexometer is well documented.

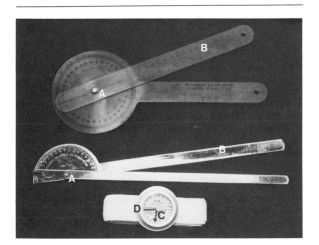

Fig. 7.2 The two instruments illustrated at the top of the photograph are examples of the conventional goniometer. The instrument below is an example of a goniometer which uses a gravity needle and a compass needle similar in principle to the flexometer. A. Axis of rotation is aligned with the joint center. B. Arms of the goniometer are aligned with the long axis of the adjacent segments. C. Gravity needle. D. Compass needle.

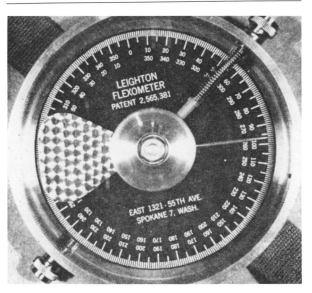

Fig. 7.3 The Leighton Flexometer or similar devices are recommended because range of motion measurements are made with respect to a fixed external reference and are recorded in degrees.

Fig. 7.4

FLEXIBILITY TEST REPORT FORM

Name _____ Sport _____

Birthdate _____ Position played _____

	Right	Left	Right	Left	Right	Left	Right	Left
Date								
Weight (kg)								
Height (cm)								
Arm length (cm)								
Leg length (cm)								
Room temperature (°C)								
Prior warm up*								
Measurements (°)								
Neck								
flexion/extension								
lateral flexion								
rotation								
Shoulder								
flexion/extension								
abduction/adduction								
rotation								
Elbow								
flexion/extension								
Radio-Ulnar								
supination/pronation								
Wrist								
flexion/extension								
Hip								
extension/flexion								
adduction/abduction								
rotation								
Knee								
flexion/extension								
Ankle								
flexion/extension								
Trunk								
lateral flexion								
rotation								
Examiner's Initials								

*Indicate no, yes passive, yes mild exercise, or yes vigorous exercise.

4. The device can measure several joints and joint actions.

5. It is relatively inexpensive compared to X-ray, photographic, or projector-type measures; it gives instant results.

6. All the reliability coefficients reported in the literature are high.

The flexometer (Cat. No. 5059) is available from:

> J.A. Preston Canada Co.
> 3220 Wharton Way
> Mississauga, Ontario
> L4X 2C1

The major problem is to identify a test protocol suitable for one's particular needs. Munroe and Romance (1975) used the Leighton flexometer to develop a battery of tests which could be used to predict overall flexibility. The four measures identified were trunk lateral flexion, shoulder ad- and abduction, hip ad- and abduction, and wrist flexion and extension. These four tests could be used to form the basic skeleton of tests to measure overall flexibility.

The coach and/or team therapist must then identify joint actions specific to the skills used in their sport and incorporate these measures into the overall procedure. The flexibility test should be administered prior to the start of the season and periodically throughout the season. Measures should be taken also following an injury and after rehabilitation.

The actual testing procedure is outlined in the eleven steps below. All information should be recorded accurately on a form similar to the one found in Figure 7.4. Subjects should be requested to wear a bathing suit if possible.

1. Check and calibrate equipment (for further details see Chapter 6): a) flexometer; b) measuring tape; c) room thermometer; d) weight scale; e) report form.

2. Record personal information: name, birthdate, sport, position played.

3. Record the date.

4. Weigh subject; record in kilograms.

5. Measure subject's height without shoes; record in centimeters.

6. Measure subject's right arm from the acromion (tip of the shoulder) to the tip of the middle finger; record in centimeters.

7. Measure subject's right leg from the greater trochanter to the floor; record in centimeters.

8. Record room temperature in degrees Celsius.

9. Indicate prior warm-up intensity.

10. Measure joint range of motion using procedures outlined by Leighton (1966). Record in degrees. See Appendix 7.1.

11. Initial appropriate space on report form.

INTERPRETATION OF RESULTS

Interpretation of these results is difficult because normal ranges of motion for athletes in different sports are not well documented in the literature. Leighton (1966) presented flexibility measures from forty sixteen-year-old boys which may be used for general comparisons. The coach and therapist, however, must be able to identify problem areas specific to their sport. From the above test results, one cannot make a prediction concerning successful performance or prevention of injury, but possibly one will be able to identify the areas that need attention.

FEE STRUCTURE

There should be no direct fee to the athletes, as the team therapist or coach could easily gain experience in the use of the flexometer. The tester should attend a course to learn to identify specific anatomical landmarks, to understand joint actions, to be introduced to the flexometer and the test protocol.

There are no calculations necessary, as the measurements are read directly from the flexometer in degrees. These measures are then recorded directly on the test report form.

REFERENCES

Adams, A. Effects of various conditioning programs on ligament strength. Report to southwest district *AAPHER* Convention, 1965.

Åstrand, P. and K. Rodahl. *Textbook of Work Physiology.* New York: McGraw-Hill Book Company, 1977.

Austin, Karin. Fall flex feature. *Canadian Cross Country Skiers Guide* 1977.

Baldwin, J. and K. Cunningham. Goniometry under attack: a clinical study involving physiotherapists. *Physiotherapy Canada.* 26(2): 74-76, 1974.

Berson, B.L., T.L. Passoff, S. Nagelberg and J. Thornton. Injury patterns in squash players. *Am. J. Sports Med.* 6(6): 323-325, 1978.

Billig, H.E. *Mobilization of the Human Body.* Palo Alto: Stanford University Press, 1941.

Boone, D., S. Azen, C. Lin, C. Spence, C. Baron and L. Lynn. Reliability of goniometric measurements. *Phys. Ther.* 58: 1355-1360, 1978.

Boone, D. and S. Azen. Normal range of motion of joints in male subjects. *J. Bone and Joint Surg.* 61-A(5): 756-760, 1979.

Broer, M.R. and N.R. Galles. Importance of relationship between various body measurements in performance of the toe-touch test. *Res. Quart.* 29: 253-263, 1958.

Burley, L.R., H.C. Dobill and B.J. Farrell. Relations of power, speed, flexibility and certain anthropometric measures of junior high school girls. *Res. Quart.* 32(4): 443-448, 1961.

Corbin, C.B., L.J. Dowell, R. Lindsey and H. Tolson. *Concepts in Physical Education.* Dubuque, Iowa: Wm. C. Brown Co. Publishers, 4th edition, 1981.

Cotten, D.J. A comparison of selected trunk flexibility tests. *Amer. Corrective Therapy J.* 26(1): 24, 1972.

Cotten, D.J. and J.S. Waters. Immediate effect of four types of warm up activities upon static flexibility of four selected joints. *Amer. Corr. Ther. J.* 24(5): 133-136, 1970.

Couch, Jean. The perfect post run stretching routine. *Runners World* 84-89, 1979.

Cureton, T.K. Flexibility as an aspect of fitness. *Res. Quart.* 12: 381-391, 1941.

deVries, H.A. Prevention of muscular distress after exercise. *Res. Quart.* 32: 177-185, 1961.

deVries, H.A. Evaluation of static stretching procedures for improvement of flexibility. *Res. Quart.* 33(2): 223-229, 1962.

deVries, H.A. The looseness factor in speed and O_2 consumption of anaerobic 100 yard dash. *Res. Quart.* 34: 305, 1963.

deVries, H.A. *Physiology of Exercise.* Dubuque, Iowa: Wm. C. Brown Co. Publishers, 2nd edition, 1974.

Dintiman, G.B. Effects of various training programs on running speed. *Res. Quart.* 25: 456, 1964.

Fieldman, H. Effects of selected extensibility exercises on the flexibility of the hip joint. *Res. Quart.* 37(3): 326-331, 1966.

Fieldman, H. Relative contribution of the back and hamstring muscles in the performance of the toe-touch test after selected extensibility exercises. *Res. Quart.* 39(3): 518-523, 1967.

Fleishman, E. Factor analysis of physical fitness tests. *Educational and Psychological Measurement* 23(4): 647-661, 1963.

Fredensborg, N. Unilateral joint laxity in unilateral congenital dislocation of the hip. *International Orthopaedics* 2: 177-178, 1978.

Glick, J.M. A study of ligamentous looseness in football players and its relation to injury. *Abbott Proc.* 1: 34-39, 1971.

Glick, J.M. Muscle strains: prevention and treatment. *Physician and Sportsmed.* 8(11): 73-77, 1980.

Grahame, R. and J.M. Jenkins. Joint hypermobility asset or liability. *Ann. Rheum. Dis.* 31: 109-111, 1972.

Grobaker, M.R. and G.A. Stull. Thermal applications as a determiner of joint flexibility. *Am. Correct Ther. J.* 29(1): 3-8, 1975.

Harris, M.L. A factor analytic study of flexibility. *Res. Quart.* 40(1): 62-70, 1969.

Harris, M.L. Flexibility. *Physical Therapy* 49(6): 591-601, 1969.

Hawkins, R.J. and J.C. Kennedy. Impingement syndrome in athletes. *Am. J. Sports Med.* 8(3): 151-158, 1980.

Holland, G.J. The physiology of flexibility. A review of the literature in *Kinesiology Review*: 49-62, 1968.

Holt, L.E. *Scientific Stretching for Sport (3S).* Halifax, N.S.: Sport Research Limited.

Holt, L.E., J.M. Travis and V. Okita. Comparative study of three stretching techniques. *Perceptual and Motor Skills* 31: 611-616, 1970.

Hupprich, F. and P.O. Sigerseth. Specificity of flexibility in girls. *Res. Quart.* 21: 25-33, 1950.

Hutchins, G.L. The relationship of selected strength and flexibility variables to antero-posterior posture of college women. *Res. Quart.* 36(3): 253-269, 1965.

Jackson, D.W., H. Jarrett, D. Bailey, J. Kausek, J. Swanson and J.W. Powell. Injury prediction in the young athlete: A preliminary report. *Am. J. Sports Med.* 6(1): 6-13, 1978.

Johns, R.J. and V. Wright. Relative importance of various tissues in joint stiffness. *J. Appl. Physiol.* 17: 824-828, 1962.

Johnson, R.J., M.H. Pope and G. Weisman *et al.* The knee injury in skiing. A multifaceted approach. *Am. J. Sports Med.* 7: 321-327, 1979.

Kalenak, A. and C.A. Morehouse. Knee stability and knee ligament injuries. *J.A.M.A.* 234(11): 1143-1145, 1975.

Karpovich, P.V. and G.P. Karpovich. Electrogoniometer: A new device for study of joints in action. *Fed. Proc.* 18: 79, 1959.

Kendall, H.A. and P. Florence Kendall. Normal flexibility according to age groups. *J. Bone and Joint Surg.* 30A: 690-694, 1949.

Kennedy, J.C. and R.J. Hawkins. Swimmer's shoulder. *Phys. and Sportsmed.* 2: 35-38, 1974.

Kennedy, J.C., R. Hawkins and W.B. Krissoff. Orthopedic manifestations of swimming. *Am. J. Sports Med.* 6: 309-322, 1978.

Klafs, C. and D. Arnheim. *Modern Principles of Athletic Training.* Saint Louis: C.V. Mosby Company, 1973.

Klein, K.K. Improving efficiency and preventing stress in joggers and distance runners. In: Terauds, J. and G.G. Dales (ed). *Sciences in Athletics*: 239-247, 1978.

Knight, K. Knee rehabilitation by the daily adjustable progressive resistive exercise technique. *Am. J. Sports Med.* 7(6): 336-337, 1979.

Kott, F.J. and M.A. Mundale. Range of mobility of the cervical spine. *Arch. Phys. Med.* 40: 379, 1959.

Kraus, H. and R. Hirschland. Minimum muscular fitness tests in school children. *Res. Quart.* 25(2): 178-187, 1954.

Kresci, Vladimir and P. Koch. *Muscle and Tendon Injuries in Athletes.* Stuttgart: Thieme Publishers, 1979.

Kuland, D.N., F.C. McCue III, D.A. Rockwell and J.H. Gieck. Tennis injuries: prevention and treatment. *Amer. J. of Sports Med.* 7(4): 249-253, 1979.

Laras, G.S., C.M. Tipton and R.R. Cooper. Influence of physical activity on ligament insertions in the knees of dogs. *J. Bone Joint Surg.* 53A: 275-286, 1971.

Laubach, L.L. and J.T. McConville. Relationships between flexibility, anthropometry and somatotype of college men. *Res. Quart.* 37(2): 241-251, 1966.

Leighton, J.R. A simple objective, and reliable measure of flexibility. *Research Quarterly,* 13: 205-216, 1942.

Leighton, J.R. Flexibility characteristics of males ten to eighteen years of age. *Arch. Phys. Med. Rehab.* 37: 494-499, 1956.

Leighton, J.R. Flexibility characteristics of four specialized skill groups of college athletes. *Arch. Phys. Med. Rehab.* 38(1): 24, 1957.

Leighton, J.R. The Leighton flexometer and flexibility test. *J.A.P.M.R.* 20(3): 86-93, 1966.

Logan, G.A. and B. Egstrom. Effects of slow and fast stretching on the sacro-femoral angle. *J. Assoc. Phys. Mental Rehab.* 15(3): 85-89, 1961.

Logan, G.A. *Adaptations of Muscular Activity.* Belmont: Wadsworth Publishing Co. Inc., 1965.

Macrae, I.F. and V. Wright. Measurement of back movement. *An. Rheum. Dis.* 28: 584-589, 1969.

Mann, R.A. and J. Hagy. Biomechanics of walking, running and sprinting. *Am. J. Sports Med.* 8(5): 345-350, 1980.

Markos, P.D. Ipsilateral and contralateral effects of proprioceptive neuromuscular facilitation technique on hip motion and electromyographic activity. *Phys. Ther.* 59(11): 1366-1373, 1979.

Marshall, J.L., N. Johanson, T.L. Wickiewicz, H.M. Tischler, B.L. Koslin, S. Zeno and A. Meyers. Joint looseness: A function of the person and the joint. *Med. Sci. in Sports and Ex.* 12(3): 189-194, 1980.

Massey, B.H. and N.L. Chaudet. Effects of systematic heavy resistance exercises on range of joint movement in young male adults. *Res. Quart.* 27(1): 41, 1956.

Mathews, D.K., V. Shaw and M. Bohnen. Hip flexibility of college women as related to length of body segments. *Res. Quart.* 28(4): 352-356, 1957.

Mathews, D.K., V. Shaw and J.B. Woods. Hip flexibility of elementary school boys as related to body segments. *Res. Quart.* 30(3): 297-302, 1959.

McCue, B.F. Flexibility measurements of college women. *Res. Quart.* 24: 316-324, 1953.

Moore, M.L. The measurement of joint motion — Part II: The techniques of goniometry. *Phys. Ther. Review* 29: 256-264, 1949.

Moore, M.A. and R.S. Hutton. Electromyographic investigation of muscle stretching techniques. *Med. Sci. in Sports and Exer.* 12(5): 322-329, 1980.

Munroe, R.A. and T.J. Romance. Use of Leighton flexometer in the development of a short flexibility test battery. *Am. Correct. Ther.* 29(1): 22-25, 1975.

Nicholas, J.A. Injuries to knee ligaments, relationship to looseness and tightness in football players. *J.A.M.A.* 212: 2236-2239, 1970.

Noyes, F.R., P.J. Torvik, W.B. Hyde and J.L. DeLucas.

Biomechanics of ligament failure. *J. Bone Joint Surg.* 56A(7): 1406-1418, 1974.

Physical Fitness Research Digest. Ed. H. Harrison Clarke, published by President's Council on Physical Fitness and Sports, Washington: 5(4): 3-21, 1975.

Rasch, P.J., R. Manescalco, W.R. Pierson and G. Logan. Effect of exercise, immobilization and intermittent stretching on strength of knee ligaments of albino rats. *J. Appl. Physiol.* 15: 289-290, 1960.

Renstrom, P. and L. Peterson. Groin injuries in athletes. *Brit. J. Sports Med.* 14: 30-36, 1980.

Richardson, A.B., F.W. Jobe and H.R. Collins. The shoulder in competitive swimming. *Am. J. Sports Med.* 8(3): 159-163, 1980.

Rigby, B.J., N. Hirai and J.O. Spikes. The mechanical properties of rat tail tendon. *J. General Physiol.* 43: 265-283, 1958.

Sigerseth, P.O. and C. Haliski. The flexibility of football players. *Res. Quart.* 21: 394-398, 1950.

Smart, G.W., J.E. Taunton and D.B. Clement. Achilles tendon disorders in runners — a review. *Med. Sci. Sports Exer.* 12(4): 231-243, 1980.

Smodlaka, V.N. Groin pain in soccer players. *Phys. and Sportsmed.* 8(8): 57-61, 1980.

Speakman, Haddan and J.S. Kung. The flexometer. *Physiotherapy Canada* 30(1): 21-23, 1978.

Tanigawa, M.C. Comparison of the hold-relax procedure and passive mobilization on increasing muscle length. *Phys. Ther.* 52(7): 725-735, 1972.

Tipton, C.M., R.D. Matthes, J.A. Maynard and R.A. Carey. The influence of physical activity on ligaments and tendons. *Med. Sci. in Sports* 7(3): 165-175, 1975.

Twomey, L. and J. Taylor. A description of two new instruments for measuring the ranges of sagittal and horizontal plane motions in the lumbar region. *Aust. J. Physiother.* 25(5): 201-203, 1979.

Tyrance, H.J. Relationship of extreme body types to ranges of flexibility. *Res. Quart.* 29(3): 349-359, 1958.

Wear, C.L. The relationship of flexibility to length of body segment. *Res. Quart.* 34: 234, 1963.

Weisman, G., M.H. Pope and R.J. Johnson. Cyclic loading in knee ligament injuries. *Am. J. Sports Med.* 8(1): 24-30, 1980.

Wells, K.F. and E.K. Dillan. The sit and reach — a test of back and leg flexibility. *Res. Quart.* 23: 115-118, 1952.

Wickstrom, R.L. The effects of low resistance, high repetition progressive resistance exercises upon selected measures of strength and flexibility. *J. Assn. for Phys. and Mental Rehab.* 14(6): 161, 1960.

Wiechec, F.J. and F.H. Krusen. A new method of joint measurement and a review of the literature. *Am. J. Surg.* 43: 3, 1979.

Wilmer, H.A. and E. Elkins. An optical goniometer for observing range of motion of joints. *Arch. of Phys. Med.* 28: 694-704, 1947.

Zankel, H.T. Photogoniometry. *Arch. of Phys. Med.* 32: 227-228, 1951.

APPENDIX 7.1

Extracts from
The Leighton Flexometer and Flexibility Test
by J.R. Leighton

Reprinted, with permission of the American Corrective Therapy Association, Inc., from the Journal of the Association of Physical and Mental Rehabilitation, Volume 20, number 3, 1966, pages 86-93.

MEASUREMENT TECHNIC

Neck

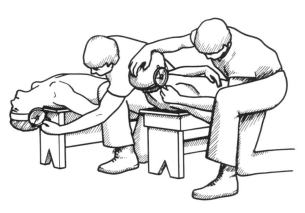

Fig. 7.5   Neck flexion and extension.

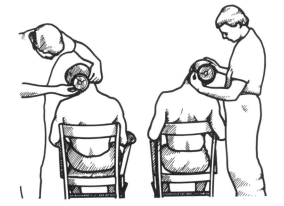

Fig. 7.6   Neck lateral flexion.

Flexion and Extension (Fig. 7.5):

Starting position

Supine position on bench, head and neck projecting over end, shoulders touching edge, arms at sides. Instrument fastened to either side of head over ear.

Movement

Count (1) head raised and moved to position as near chest as possible, dial locked (2) head lowered and moved to position as near end of bench as possible, pointer locked (3) subject relaxes, reading taken.

Caution

Shoulders may not be raised from bench during flexion, nor back unduly arched during extension. Buttocks and shoulders must remain on bench during movement.

Lateral Flexion (Fig. 7.6):

Starting position

Sitting position in low-backed armchair, back straight, hands grasping chair arms, upper arms hooked over back of chair. Instrument fastened to back of head.

Movement

Count (1) head moved in arc sideward left as far as possible, dial locked (2) head moved in arc sideward right as far as possible, pointer locked (3) subject relaxes, reading taken.

Caution

Position in chair may not be changed during movement. Shoulders may not be raised or lowered.

Rotation (Fig. 7.7):

Starting position

Supine position on bench, head and neck projecting over, shoulders touching edge and arms at sides of bench. Instrument fastened to top of head.

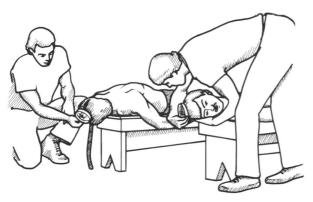

Fig. 7.7 Neck rotation.

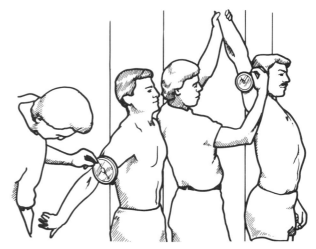

Fig. 7.8 Shoulder flexion and extension.

Movement

Count (1) head turned left as far as possible, dial locked (2) head turned right as far as possible, pointer locked (3) subject relaxes, reading taken.

Caution

Shoulders may not be raised from bench.

Shoulder

Flexion and Extension (Fig. 7.8):

Starting position

Standing position at projecting corner of wall, arm to be measured extending just beyond projecting corner, arms at sides, back to wall, shoulder blades, buttocks and heels touching wall. Instrument fastened to side of upper arm.

Movement

Count (1) arm moved forward and upward in an arc as far as possible, palm of hand sliding against wall, dial locked (2) arm moved downward and backward in an arc as far as possible, palm of hand sliding against wall, pointer locked (3) subject relaxes, reading taken.

Caution

Heels, buttocks and shoulders must touch wall at all times during movement. Elbow of arm being measured must be kept straight. Palm of hand of arm being measured must be against wall when dial and pointer are locked.

Adduction and Abduction (Fig. 7.9):

Starting position

Standing position with arms at sides, left (right) side of body towards wall, shoulder touching same, left (right) fist doubled with knuckles forward, thumb-side of fist touching hip and opposite side of fist touching wall, feet together, knees and elbows straight. Instrument fastened to back of right (left) upper arm.

Movement

Count (1) palm of right (left) hand pressed against side of leg, dial locked (2) arm moved sideward, outward and upward in an arc as far as possible, pointer locked (3) subject relaxes, reading taken.

Caution

Left (right) fist must be kept in contact with the body and wall at all times. Knees, body and elbows must be kept straight throughout movement. Arm must be raised directly sideward, not forward or backward. Heels of feet may not be raised from floor.

Rotation (Fig. 7.10):

Starting position

Standing position at projecting corner of wall, arm to be measured extended sideward and bent

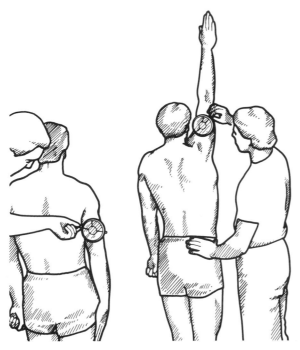

Fig. 7.9   Shoulder adduction and abduction.

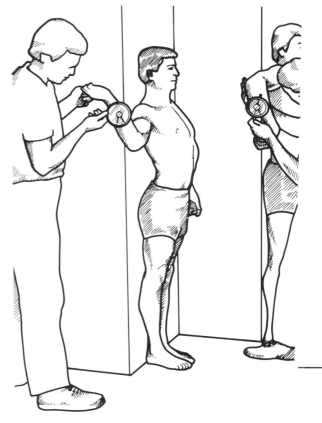

Fig. 7.10   Shoulder rotation.

to right angle at elbow, shoulder extended just beyond projecting corner, opposite arm at side of body, back to wall, shoulder blades, buttocks and heels touching wall. Instrument fastened to side of forearm.

Movement

Count (1) forearm moved downward and backward in an arc as far as possible, dial locked (2) forearm moved forward, upward and backward in arc as far as possible, pointer locked (3) subject relaxes, reading taken.

Caution

Upper arm being measured must be held directly sideward and parallel with the floor during movement. Heels, buttocks, and shoulders must touch wall at all times.

Elbow

Flexion and Extension (Fig. 7.11):

Starting position

Squatting or sitting position facing table or bench with upper portion of arm being measured

resting back down across nearest table corner so that the elbow extends just beyond one edge and the armpit is resting against the adjacent edge. Instrument fastened to back of wrist.

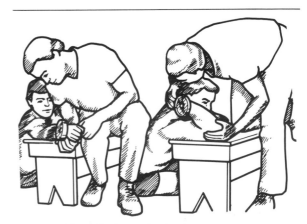

Fig. 7.11   Elbow flexion and extension.

Movement

Count (1) wrist moved upward and backward in an arc to position as near shoulder as possible, dial locked (2) wrist moved forward and downward until arm is forcibly extended, pointer locked (3) subject relaxes, reading taken.

Caution

Upper arm may not be tilted or moved during measurement.

Radial-Ulnar

Supination and Pronation (Fig. 7.12):

Starting position

Sitting position in standard armchair, back straight, forearms resting on chair arms, fists doubled and extended beyond ends of chair arms, wrist of arm to be measured held straight. Strap is grasped in hand, fastening instrument to front of fist. (Common chair and table of suitable height may be substituted for armchair.)

Movement

Count (1) thumb-side of fist turned outward and downward as far as possible, dial locked (2) thumb-side of fist turned upward, downward and inward as far as possible, pointer locked (3) subject relaxes, reading taken.

Caution

Body and forearm must remain stationary, except for specified movement, throughout measurement. No leaning of the body may be permitted.

Wrist

Flexion and Extension (Fig. 7.13):

Starting position

Standing position in standard armchair, back straight, forearms resting on chair arms, fists doubled and extended beyond ends of chair arms, palm of hand to be measured turned up. Instrument fastened to thumbside of fist. (Common chair and table of suitable height may be substituted for armchair.)

Movement

Count (1) fist moved upward and backward in an arc as far as possible, dial locked (2) fist moved forward, downward and backward in an arc as far as possible, pointer locked (3) subject relaxes, reading taken.

Caution

Forearm may not be raised from chair arm during movement.

Hip

Extension and Flexion (Fig. 7.14):

Starting position

Standing position, feet together, knees stiff, arms extended above head, hands clasped with palms up. Instrument fastened to either side of hip at height of umbilicus.

Movement

Count (1) bend backward as far as possible, dial

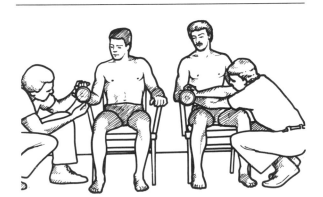

Fig. 7.12 Radial-ulnar supination and pronation.

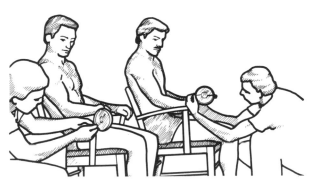

Fig. 7.13 Wrist flexion and extension.

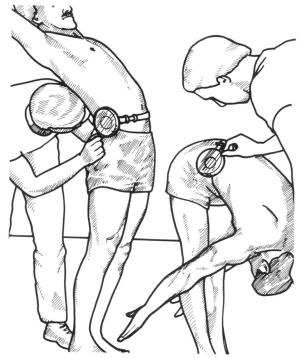

Fig. 7.14   Hip extension and flexion.

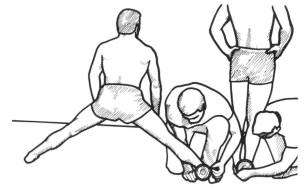

Fig. 7.15   Hip adduction and abduction.

locked (2) bend forward as far as possible, pointer locked (3) subject relaxes, reading taken.

Caution

Knees may not be bent but must remain straight throughout movement. Feet may not be shifted. Toes and heels may not be raised.

Adduction and Abduction (Fig. 7.15):

Starting position

Standing position, feet together, knees straight, arms at side. Instrument fastened to back of either leg.

Movement

Count (1) starting position, dial locked (2) leg to which instrument is not attached is moved sideward as far as possible, pointer locked (3) subject relaxes, reading taken.

Caution

Body must remain in upright position throughout movement. Knees must be kept straight with the feet assuming a position on line and parallel.

Rotation (Fig. 7.16):

Starting position

Sitting position on bench with left (right) leg resting on and foot projecting over end of bench, knee straight, right (left) leg extending downward, foot resting on floor. Instrument fastened to bottom of left (right) foot.

Movement

Count (1) left (right) foot turned outward as far as possible, dial locked (2) left (right) foot turned inward as far as possible, pointer locked (3) subject relaxes, reading taken.

Caution

Knee and ankle joints must remain locked throughout movement. Position of hips may not be changed during measurement.

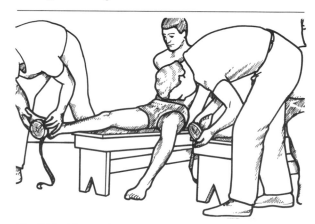

Fig. 7.16   Hip rotation.

Knee

Flexion and Extension (Fig. 7.17):

Starting position

Prone position on box or bench with knees at end of and lower legs extending beyond end of bench, arms at sides of and hands grasping edges of bench. Instrument fastened to outside of either ankle.

Movement

Count (1) foot moved upward and backward in an arc to position as near buttocks as possible, dial locked (2) foot moved forward and downward until leg is forcibly extended, pointer locked (3) subject relaxes, reading taken.

Caution

Position of upper leg may not be changed during movement.

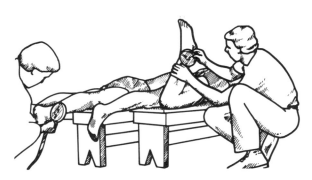

Fig. 7.17   Knee flexion and extension.

Ankle

Flexion and Extension (Fig. 7.18):

Starting position

Sitting position on bench with left (right) leg resting on and foot projecting over end of bench, knee straight, right (left) leg extending downward, foot resting on floor. Instrument fastened to inside of left (right) foot.

Movement

Count (1) left (right) foot turned downward as far as possible, dial locked (2) left (right) foot turned

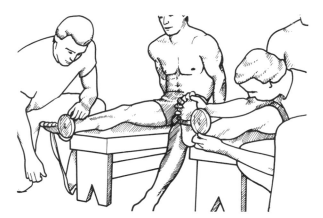

Fig. 7.18   Ankle flexion and extension.

upward and toward the knee as far as possible, pointer locked (3) subject relaxes, reading taken.

Caution

Knee of leg being measured must be kept straight throughout movement. No sideward turning of the foot may be allowed.

Inversion and Eversion (Fig. 7.19):

Starting position

Sitting on end of bench, knees projecting over and lower legs downward with calves resting against end board. Shoes (low cut) should be worn. Instrument fastened to front of foot.

Movement

Count (1) foot turned inward as far as possible, dial locked (2) foot turned outward as far as possi-

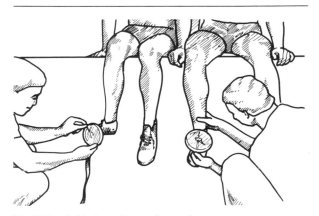

Fig. 7.19   Ankle inversion and eversion.

ble, pointer locked (3) subject relaxes, reading taken.

Caution

Position of lower leg may not be changed during measurement.

Trunk

Lateral Flexion (Fig. 7.20):

Starting position

Standing position, feet together, knees straight, arms at sides. Instrument fastened to middle of back at nipple height.

Movement

Count (1) bend sidewards to the left as far as possible, dial locked (2) bend sidewards to the right as far as possible, pointer locked (3) subject relaxes, reading taken.

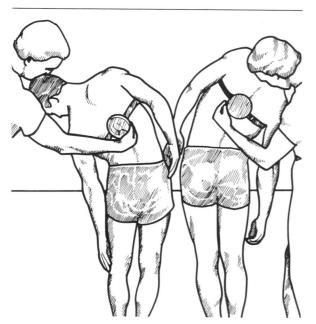

Fig. 7.20   Trunk lateral flexion.

Caution

Both feet must remain flat on floor, heels may not be raised during measurement. Knees must be kept straight throughout movement. Subject may bend sidewards and backwards but must not be allowed to bend forward.

Rotation (Fig. 7.21):

Starting position

Supine position on bench, legs together, knees raised above hips, lower legs parallel to bench and body. Assistant holds subject's shoulders. Instrument fastened to middle rear of upper legs, strap going around both legs.

Movement

Count (1) knees lowered to the left as far as possible, dial locked (2) knees brought back to starting position and lowered to the right as far as possible, pointer locked (3) subject relaxes, reading taken.

Caution

Subject's shoulders must not be permitted to rise from the bench during movement. Knees must be moved directly sidewards at the height of the hips, not above or below.

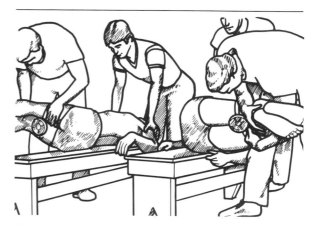

Fig. 7.21   Trunk rotation.

CHAPTER EIGHT | Field Tests

A. Reed

INTRODUCTION

The previous chapters have dealt with the evaluation of specific physiological components in a controlled laboratory environment. In many instances, it also is possible to obtain objective and reliable measures in competitive conditions. Such testing situations are no less "scientific" than, and may be just as rigorously controlled as, the more traditional laboratory tests.

What Is A Field Test?

A field test is a test which is conducted in an environment which attempts to simulate the actual competitive situation. Thus, the measurement of VO_2 max of a rower running on the treadmill is *not* a field test. The measurement of VO_2 max of this rower on a rowing ergometer in the laboratory is also *not* a field test. The measurement of VO_2 max while rowing over water in the course of a performance trial *is* a field test.

The Role of the Field Test

Results which are gained on a proper field test should be considered as complementary to those obtained through traditional laboratory tests, and neither should be considered as a replacement for the other. Most athletes undergo various stages of preliminary background training leading up to a sport-specific training stage. It is in this latter phase of training that field testing is most beneficial. Field test results are of most practical significance when they are used for comparison with results for the same individual on repeated tests, rather than for comparison with results of a larger reference group.

The development of good field tests is in its infancy. Nevertheless, by adhering to proper criteria, and with a little innovation, quality field tests may be developed and modified for practically any sport or activity.

CRITERIA FOR EVALUATION OF FIELD TESTS

Validity

A test is valid when it actually measures what it claims to measure. Field tests, like all other tests, must be validated. The way in which this is done, however, may be unique. Since the purpose of the field test is to get some physiological measurements in the simulated competitive situation, it is necessary to establish the validity of at least the following two factors:

1. the simulation of the performance
2. the selection of the physiological measurements.

Validating the Simulation

In order to assess whether a field test protocol accurately reflects the demands of the competitive situation, some form of analysis of the target performance must be undertaken. The result of such an analysis then forms the basis of the protocol. Since actual performance often varies from intended performance, some form of measurement of performance factors during the actual test must be taken and compared to the intended performance demanded by the protocol. Thus, the following criteria are suggested for establishing the validity of the field test simulation:

1. Field test protocols should be based upon a thorough analysis of the target performance to be simulated.
2. Field test protocols should include sufficient performance measurements to allow comparison of test performance to the target performance analysis upon which the protocol was based.

These two criteria establish the principle that field tests are developed by starting with a target performance analysis and then proceeding to the test design. They also establish the principle that field tests have both performance and physiological measurements. The performance measurements reveal the quality of the simulated effort, and the physiological measurements provide some insights into the physical basis of the performance.

A thorough analysis of the target performance would be one which considers the *temporal*, *movement*, and *environmental* factors of the athletic performance. Thus, some form of time-motion study combined with measurement of environmental factors could be used to establish the "thoroughness" of the performance analysis.

For example, a 400-meter time trial could be a target performance for freestyle swimming. A sample of 400-meter races at the target level of competition could be analyzed to establish a temporal pattern by split times, a movement pattern by stroke rates, and relevant environmental factors like water temperature, pool dimensions, etc. Criterion #1 suggests that these data form the basis of the performance protocol of a 400-meter freestyle swim field test.

Similarly, in a team sport like ice hockey, analysis of shift times into sprinting and gliding-type skating segments, combined with analysis of movement patterns such as the amount of forward, lateral, diagonal, or circular skating, could be used to identify a test skating pattern that is reasonably representative of the skating demands at a particular competitive level. Environmental factors such as rink dimensions, equipment worn during the test, etc., would also form part of the test protocol in keeping with Criterion #1.

In both examples, Criterion #2 would require that performance measurements such as split times or skate pattern times be included along with physiological measurements to validate that the intended simulation actually happened.

Validating the Selection of Physiological Measurements

The major factor that separates a field test from a time trial, dry run, scrimmage, or some other type of sports simulation activity is the measurement of physiological function. These measurements give some insight into the physical basis of the performance, so that judgments can be made about what physiological factor(s) might best be related to the performance. This often has been called "identifying the weak link". These measurements also can verify the effectiveness of programs aimed at specific physiological training effects.

The selection of physiological measurements should be rationalized on a proven relationship between the factor being measured and the target performance. This relationship will not be a simple cause-effect, since it is assumed that sports performance is too complex to be explained by any single factor. Selection of such measurements, however, should be restricted to those which are sensitive and responsive to the fluctuations in performance. This implies that previous research studies will have to point the way to which physiological measurements meet this requirement. It also would be useful to give priority to measurement of physiological responses that are known to be sensitive to training. This will increase the value of the field test as a monitor of training. Physiological responses often are included as indicators of intensity of effort. Intermittent-type performance is clearly affected by the type and amount of recovery between work intervals, so that measurements of recovery processes would be relevant in field tests for those sports. Thus, the following criteria are suggested for the selection of physiological measurements:

3. Physiological measurements should be limited to those which are known to be sensitive and responsive to the training for, and execution of, the target performance upon which the field test is based.

4. Physiological measurements should be used to monitor the intensity of effort in field tests.

5. Physiological measurements of recovery processes should be used in field tests of intermittent sports.

Reliability

A test is reliable when the results are consistent and reproducible. Field tests also should be reliable. It is assumed that the environmental factors are under less control in the field than in the lab. This implies that when standard test-retest procedures are used to establish the reliability of a field test, the conditions under which the simulated performance was repeated must be identified carefully. In some situations, the time between test-retest procedures may be longer than the usual few days, due to unfavorable field conditions, e.g., wind velocity, water conditions, etc. These factors, however, do not preclude, but only modify, the use of the test-retest procedure to establish field test reliability.

Using test-retest procedures, the reliability of a given field test should be established over a reasonable range of environmental conditions so as not to overly restrict its use.

Also, field test results should be independent of the personnel conducting the test. This can be established easily by having different test administrators for some of the test-retest procedures. Generating standardized test instructions will help minimize the influence of the test administrator.

Thus the following criteria are suggested for establishing reliability:

6. Reliability of field tests should be established by standard test-retest procedures.

7. The conditions under which the reliability of the field test was established should be identified carefully.

8. Field tests should be used under environmental conditions similar to those under which their reliability was established.

9. Where possible, field test reliability should be established over a range of environmental situations.

10. Field test objectivity should be established by standard test-retest procedures using different test administrators.

Summary

Ten criteria have been identified as guidelines for the evaluation of field tests of fitness. The criteria suggest the basis of test validity, reliability, and objectivity. The validity criteria focus on the basis of the performance simulation in the field and the selection of the physiological measurements. The reliability and objectivity criteria focus on the application of test-retest methods to the environmental factors involved in field testing of fitness.

The effective field test is one which applies these criteria to a specific sport situation.

Evaluating The Health Status of The Athlete

R. Backus

INTRODUCTION

The SPORT MEDICINE COUNCIL OF CANADA (SMCC) has developed a report form for physicians to follow when assessing the health status of athletes. Where variation or controversy exists in the protocols used for assessment, a recommended procedure has been outlined. Although condensed proformas have been published (Smilkstein, 1981), this comprehensive assessment form will offer the elite athlete a more thorough clinical evaluation.

An excellent rationale has been documented (Sapega and Nicholas, 1981) for using musculoskeletal profiling for orthopaedic assessments. It advocates the use of bilateral baseline data and more sophisticated instrumentation (e.g., Cybex isokinetic dynamometers) where possible, and suggests the clinical applications. The intent of the attached SMCC documents, however, is to permit standardized assessments of musculo-skeletal status without expensive instrumentation.

The use of hematology in the assessment of health status for the elite athlete deserves special mention. Williamson (1981) has suggested that borderline "sports anemia" associated primarily with distance events is an adaptive response to maximize oxygen transport. If other forms of anemia can be excluded on the clinical work-up, no treatment is necessary. Even if hemoglobin levels are normal, Clement and Asmundson (1982) suggest that a latent iron deficiency is common in endurance athletes and that serum ferritin should routinely be monitored in addition to hemoglobin levels. Their work suggests that the primary cause in females is an iron deficient diet, whereas the primary cause in males is hemolysis as reflected by reduced haptoglobin levels. Ehn et al. (1980) have suggested also that low dietary intake of organic iron, as well as increased elimination, may elicit depressed iron levels in males.

The standardized procedures prepared by Dr. Richard Backus follow the SMCC reporting forms, and are to be used in conjunction with the appropriate sections on the indicated form.

SPORT MEDICINE COUNCIL OF CANADA FORMS

Available from:
Sport Medicine Council of Canada
333 River Road
Vanier, Ontario
K1L 8H9

STANDARDIZED PROCEDURES FOR ASSESSING THE HEALTH STATUS OF ATHLETES

Note: The lettering and numbering in this section refer to the letters and numbers on the Athlete Medical History Profile, starting with *Physical Examination* on page 147.

1. Central Nervous System
   Central nervous system should be assessed according to standard medical practice.
2. Ears, Eyes, Nose and Throat
   a. Ears
      (2) Drums
         Check the eardrum mobility with the Valsalva maneuver.
5. Cardiovascular
   b. Blood Pressure
      If it is elevated over 120/80 mm of mercury, retake after fifteen minutes of rest or after hyperventilation (five breaths as deeply and as quickly as possible).
8. Musculo-skeletal System
   The following is a list against which any suspected limitation of range of movement may be checked (Heck et al., 1978). "Abnor-

mal" is not used here in the usual sense; rather, it refers to a restriction of movement which, for sport purposes, it is worthwhile for the physician to note.

a. Back
  (1) Cervical
      Flexion and extension are usually designated by degrees.

      Flexion and extension: 90% from the vertical is considered normal.

      Lateral bend: placement of the ear to the shoulder on either side is considered normal.

      Rotation: 90° in either direction, or placement of the chin to the shoulder is considered normal.

  (2) Thoracic
      Flexion: initially observe any flattening of the thoracic or lumbar spine. Then, lay tape from S1 to C7 and measure in upright and fully flexed positions. There should be significant increase in length (roughly 10 cm increase is considered normal).

      Lateral bending: determine the degrees of lateral inclination of the trunk. Less than 30° is considered abnormal.

      Extension: is measured with the patient lying prone with the back and neck extended. If the angle of S1 to C7 is less than 20°, it is considered abnormal.

      Rotation: if the angle from the shoulder plane to the pelvic plane is less than 40°, it is considered abnormal.

  (5) Coccyx
      If, by rectal examination, there is no movement, it is considered abnormal.

b. Pelvis
      If there is pain, or any detectable movement at the symphysis pubis, it is considered abnormal.

c. Joints–flexibility
  (1) Shoulder
      If forward flexion is less than 140°, it is considered abnormal.

      If abduction is less than 160°, it is considered abnormal.

      If internal rotation is less than 90°, it is considered abnormal.

      If external rotation is less than 40°, it is considered abnormal.

  (2) Elbow
      If flexion is less than 135°, it is considered abnormal.

      If extension is less than 0°, it is considered abnormal.

  Forearm
      If pronation is less than 70°, it is considered abnormal.

      If supination is less than 80°, it is considered abnormal.

  (3) Wrist
      If extension is less than 60°, it is considered abnormal.

      If flexion is less than 70°, it is considered abnormal.

      If ulnar deviation is less than 30°, it is considered abnormal.

      If radial deviation is less than 15°, it is considered abnormal.

  Thumb
      If abduction is less than 50°, it is considered abnormal.

  (5) Hip
      If flexion is less than 100°, it is considered abnormal.

      If extension is less than 10°, it is considered abnormal.

      If abduction is less than 40°, it is considered abnormal.

      If adduction is less than 20°, it is considered abnormal.

  (6) Knee
      If flexion is less than 120°, it is considered abnormal.

      If hyperextension or recurvatum occurs greater than 0°, it is considered abnormal.

      Iliotibial band: Ober's test
      "The patient lies on his side with the thigh of the unaffected leg next to the table and flexed enough to obliterate any lumbar lordosis. The affected knee is then flexed to a right angle and the leg is grasped tightly with one hand while the pelvis is stabilized by the other. Then the hip is abducted widely and extended so that the thigh is in line with the body to catch the iliotibial band on the greater trochanter, maximizing its excursion. The leg is then brought towards the table in adduction. If any iliotibial band shortening is present, the hip will remain passively abducted in direct proportion to the amount of shortening." (Noble et al., 1982).

If the medial femoral condyle of the affected knee will not reach the level of the medial femoral condyle of the unaffected knee, there is iliotibial band tightening.

Hamstrings: with the patient supine and the hip in 90° of flexion, extend the knee. If it doesn't reach 0°, it is abnormal. (Measure the number of degrees from full extension of the knee.)

Quadriceps: with the patient supine, the knee should be passively flexed so that the bulk of the gastrocnemius presses firmly against the bulk of the hamstring. Anything less than this should be measured in degrees of knee flexion.

(7) Ankle

If plantar flexion is less than 40°, it is considered abnormal.

If dorsiflexion is less than 10°, it is considered abnormal.

Gastrocnemius: passive foot dorsiflexion of less than 10° with the knee in extension indicates gastrocnemius shortening in the absence of soleus shortening.

Soleus: passive foot dorsiflexion of less than 10° with the knee flexed is indicative of soleus shortening.

Great toe

An extension of less than 30° is considered abnormal.

d. Alignment

(1) Knee

i) varus: with the patient standing with the medial malleoli together, the femoral intercondylar distance should not exceed 4 cm.

ii) valgus: with the patient standing with medial femoral condyles together, the intermalleolar distance should not exceed 1 cm.

iii) recurvatum: hyperextension of the knee while standing should not exceed 0°.

(2) Patella

i) the Q angle is measured from the anterior superior iliac spine to the center of the patella to the center of the tibial tubercle and should not exceed 10°.

ii) squint is an abnormal prominence of the medial portion of the patella while standing with the feet together. This is diagnosed only by clinical judgment.

(3) Tibia

i) varum: with the athlete standing and the medial malleoli together, measure the angle of the tibia compared to vertical. If the angle is 7° or more, it is considered abnormal.

iii) torsion: with the patient lying prone, flex the knee to 90°, and compare the angle that the foot makes to the thigh. A range of 0°-15° is normal.

(4) Foot

Assess the neutral position of the foot by having the patient lie prone with the knee extended. Place the finger and thumb of one examining hand in the hollows over the neck of the talus on either side of the anterior portion of the ankle. Using the other examining hand, grasp the heads of the fourth and fifth metatarsals and rock back and forth until the talus lies centered between the fingers. This will be approximately mid-position of movement for the os calcis. Measure the number of degrees that the line of os calcis makes with the line of the tibia. If the angle is greater than 5° or less than 0° varus, it is considered abnormal.

While maintaining the above position, measure the angle the forefoot makes with regard to the perpendicular of the line of the os calcis. A forefoot varus greater than 2° or less than 0° is considered abnormal (Clement and Taunton, 1980).

(5) Leg Length

A rough estimation can be made with the patient lying prone and body in straight alignment. Look for gross differences in the level of malleoli. If there is any noticeable difference, measure the difference from the iliac crest to the lateral malleolus on both sides.

11. Laboratory studies

a. Urinalysis — complete

(1) S.G.

Urinalysis must be carried out on a morning specimen with no workout in the preceding 24 hours.

(2) Albumin

1+ or greater albumin requires a quantitative 24-hour urine for protein analysis with no workout in the preceding 48 hours.

(3) Glucose

Any glucose requires a 3-hour glucose tolerance test after three days of carbohydrate loading and no workouts.

(4) Microscopic

Presence of greater than 4 red blood cells per high power field should suggest pre- and post-workout urinalysis. Any post-workout increase in the number of red blood cells per high power field should result in workup for athletic pseudo-nephropathy (Blacklock, 1979).

b. Hematology

No workout in the preceding 24 hours should occur when doing hematology.

It should include range of normals for the laboratory carrying out the work and specify the method used if it deviates from the normal. The athletes should also avoid anti-inflammatories and any other medications for the preceding four days.

See Clement and Asmundson (1982) for rationale for additional assessment of serum ferritin.

c. Blood Chemistry

The recommended assays are the SMA12, which requires fasting for the preceding eight hours. No alcohol and no workout in the preceding 36 hours is also recommended.

13. Optional Examinations

a. Chest X-ray
b. EEG
c. EKG (resting)
d. EKG (stress)

The original tracings should be included in the report.

REFERENCES

Blacklock, N.J. Bladder trauma in the long distance runner. *Amer. J. Sports Med.* 7(4):239, 1979.

Clement, D.B., J. Taunton. A guide to the prevention of running injuries, *Can. Fam. Phys.* 26:543, 1980.

Clement, D.B., R.C. Asmundson. Nutritional intake and hematological parameters in endurance runners. *Phys. Sports Med.* 10(3):37-43, 1982.

Ehn, L., B. Carlmark, S. Hoglund. Iron status in athletes involved in intense physical activity. *Med. Sci. Sports Exercise.* 12(1):61-64, 1980.

Heck, C.V., O.E. Hendryson, C.R. Rowe. Joint motion: method of measuring and recording. In *American Academy of Orthopedic Surgeons.* London, Churchill Livingstone, 1978.

Noble, H.B., M.R. Hajek, M. Porter. Diagnosis and treatment of ilio-tibial band tightness in runners. *Phys. Sports Med.* 10(4):67-74, 1982.

Sapega, A.A., J.A. Nicholas. The use of musculo-skeletal profiling in orthopedic sportsmedicine. *Phys. Sports Med.* 9(4):80-88, 1981.

Smilkstein, G. Health evaluation of high school athletes. *Phys. Sports Med.* 9(8):73-80, 1981.

Williams, M.R. Anemia in runners and other athletes, *Phys. Sports Med.* 9(6):73-79, 1981.

513-3A

 SPORT MEDICINE COUNCIL OF CANADA
MEDICAL HISTORY INJURY REPORTING SYSTEM

ATHLETE HEALTH QUESTIONNAIRE

This form is to be completed by the athlete or in the case of minors, by the parent or guardian.

DATE _____

NAME _____
            Surname   Given Names

MALE __   FEMALE __   DATE OF BIRTH _____
                                             Month   Day   Year

HOME ADDRESS _____
             _____
             _____

HOME TELEPHONE (___) _____   BUSINESS TELEPHONE (___) _____

MARRIED __   SEPARATED __   DIVORCED __   WIDOWED __   SINGLE __

SPORT _____   EVENT _____

PASSPORT NO. _____   S.I.N. _____

Provincial Medical Insurance No. _____   Province of Registration _____

FAMILY PHYSICIAN'S NAME _____   Tel. No. (___) _____

FAMILY PHYSICIAN'S ADDRESS _____

FAMILY DENTIST'S NAME _____   Tel. No. (___) _____

FAMILY DENTIST'S ADDRESS _____

DATE OF LAST MEDICAL EXAMINATION _____

ALLERGIES _____

MEDICATIONS _____
             _____

    Please list all medications, prescription and non-prescription drugs, which you are
    presently taking.

IN CASE OF EMERGENCY, PLEASE NOTIFY:

NAME _____

ADDRESS _____

TELEPHONE NO. _____   RELATIONSHIP _____

FAMILY HISTORY

Please check the medical conditions applicable to any one of your close family members in the chart below.

	Close Family	Relation		Close Family	Relation
Allergies or Asthma			Emotional Problems		
Anemia			Kidney/ Bladder Disorder		
High Blood Pressure			Stomach Disorder		
Cancer or Tumor			Genetic Disorder		
Diabetes			Has anyone in your family under age 50 died suddenly?		
Epilepsy					
Heart Trouble					
Migraine Headaches					

Confidential When Completed

A. <u>MEDICAL</u>

Answer all questions carefully.
For "yes" answers, elaborate in the
MEDICAL CHART which follows on page 5.

1. Do you at present time
   experience:

   a) Difficulties with your eyes,
      or problems with vision?   No ___   Yes ___

   b) Difficulties with you nose
      or throat?   No ___   Yes ___

   c) Problems with hearing?   No ___   Yes ___

   d) Headaches, dizziness,
      weakness, fainting, any
      problems with coordination
      or balance?   No ___   Yes ___

   e) Numbness in any part of
      the body?   No ___   Yes ___

   f) Any tendency to shake or
      tremble?   No ___   Yes ___

   g) Cough, shortness of breath,
      chest pain or palpitations?   No ___   Yes ___

   h) Poor appetite, vomiting,
      abdominal pain, abnormal
      bowel habits?   No ___   Yes ___

   j) Any symptoms referrable to
      the urinary system?   No ___   Yes ___

   k) Any symptoms referrable to
      the muscles, bones or joints,
      i.e. stiffness, swelling,
      pain?   No ___   Yes ___

   l) Any problems with the skin
      such as sores, rashes, itchy
      or burning sensation, etc.?   No ___   Yes ___

   m) Other symptoms?   No ___   Yes ___

2. Have any of the above symptoms
   been a problem in the past?   No ___   Yes ___

3. Have you ever had, or been
   told you had, or consulted a
   physician for:

   a) Diabetes, goiter or any
      disease of the glands
      (i.e. mononucleosis)?   No ___   Yes ___

   b) Epilepsy?   No ___   Yes ___

   c) Nervous Disorder or any
      diseases of the brain or
      nervous system?   No ___   Yes ___

   d) Heart trouble or rheumatic
      fever?   No ___   Yes ___

   e) Varicose veins, phlebitis,
      hemorrhoids or any disease
      of the circulatory system?   No ___   Yes ___

B. <u>TRAUMA</u>

For "yes" answers, elaborate in the TRAUMA CHART
which follows on page 5.

1. Have you ever been treated for
   calcium deposits?   No ___   Yes ___

2. If yes, where were these deposits?
   _____

3. Have you ever experienced an
   injury to your left or right
   shoulder, arm, elbow, wrist,
   hand? Specify in Trauma Chart.   No ___   Yes ___

   If the answer to question 3 is yes answer
   questions 4-7, otherwise proceed to question 8.

4. If answer to question 3 is yes,
   did the injury incapacitate you
   for a week or longer?   No ___   Yes ___

5. Did you seek the advice or care
   of a physician, therapist,
   chiropractor or other?   No ___   Yes ___

   (Please specify the Professional.)
   _____

6. Have you ever been advised to
   have surgery to correct the
   condition? Specify in Trauma
   Chart.   No ___   Yes ___

7. Has the recommended surgery
   been completed?   No ___   Yes ___
   Date: _____

8. Have you ever had an injury
   to your head, cervical spine,
   thoracic spine (ribs), lumbar
   spine, sacroiliac joints?   No ___   Yes ___

9. If answer to question 8 is yes,
   did you seek the care of a
   physician, therapist,
   chiropractor or other?   No ___   Yes ___

   (Please specify the Professional.)
   _____

10. Do you experience pain in
    your back?   No ___   Yes ___

11. If yes, when?
    Very seldom ___   Frequently ___
    Occasionally ___
    Only after vigorous exercise ___

12. Have you ever had an injury to
    your left or right hip, knee,
    ankle, foot? Specify in Trauma
    Chart.   No ___   Yes ___

    If answer to question 12 is yes answer
    questions 13-16; otherwise proceed to
    question 17 under Trauma.

13. If answer to question 12 is yes
    did the injury incapacitate you
    for a week or longer?   No ___   Yes ___

A. MEDICAL (Con't)

    f) Any disease of the blood, easy bruising or bleeding tendency?   No ___ Yes ___

    g) Tuberculosis, asthma, or any lung disease or respiratory disorder?   No ___ Yes ___

    h) Ulcers or any disease of the stomach, intestines, liver or gall bladder?   No ___ Yes ___

    j) Sugar, albumin or blood in the urine or any disease of the kidneys or genito-urinary organs?   No ___ Yes ___

    k) Arthritis, rheumatism or any injury or disease of the bones, peripheral joints, back or spine? Specify in Medical Chart.   No ___ Yes ___

    l) Hernia or any disease of the muscles or skin?   No ___ Yes ___

    m) Cancer, tumor or growth of any kind?   No ___ Yes ___

4. Have you ever had any operations? Specify in Medical Chart.   No ___ Yes ___

5. Have you ever been advised to have a surgical operation which has not been performed? Specify in Medical Chart.   No ___ Yes ___

6. Have you ever had a head injury causing severe dizziness, loss of memory, vomiting, unconsciousness, or requiring medical attention or hospitalization?   No ___ Yes ___

7. Heat Disorder

    a) Have you ever had trouble with dehydration? (excess loss of salt and water)   No ___ Yes ___

    b) Have you ever had heat stroke? (failure of body's heat regulating system resulting in body temp. above 40.5°C (105°F)   No ___ Yes ___

    c) If yes, were you hospitalized for heat stroke?   No ___ Yes ___

    d) Other Heat Disorder? Specify in Medical Chart.   No ___ Yes ___

8. Have you ever been under observation or treatment in any hospital, sanitorium or other similar institutions? (excluding items noted under Medical question #4.)   No ___ Yes ___

B. TRAUMA (Con't)

14. Did you seek the advice of a physician, therapist, chiropractor or other?   No ___ Yes ___

    Please specify the Professional.
    _____

15. Have you ever been advised to have surgery to correct the condition? Specify in Trauma Chart.   No ___ Yes ___

16. Has the recommended surgery been completed? Date: _____   No ___ Yes ___

17. Have you ever been told that you injured the cartilage (meniscus) of either knee joint?   No ___ Yes ___

18. Do you have problems with your knee caps (patella)? i.e. chondromalacia, dislocation,etc.   No ___ Yes ___

19. Have you ever been told that you injured the ligaments of either knee joint?   No ___ Yes ___

20. Have you ever been told you have a "trick knee"?   No ___ Yes ___

21. Have you ever experienced a severe sprain of either ankle?   No ___ Yes ___

22. Do you have a pin, screw or plate somewhere in your body as a result of bone or joint surgery? Specify in Trauma Chart.   No ___ Yes ___

23. Have you ever had a bone graft or a spinal fusion?   No ___ Yes ___

    If so, where? _____
    Specify in Trauma Chart.

24. Have you had a fracture during the past two years?   No ___ Yes ___

    If so, where? _____
    _____

A. MEDICAL (Con't)

9. Have you within the last five years had any illness, disease or injury that is not included in the above?   No ___ Yes ___

10. Do you now have any deformity or physical defect?   No ___ Yes ___

11. Has your weight changed in the last year?   No ___ Yes ___

    If yes, Gain ___ kg
            Loss ___ kg

12. Any explanation for this weight change? Specify in Medical Chart.   No ___ Yes ___

13. Are you more thirsty than usual lately?   No ___ Yes ___

14. Are you involved in a sport based on weight class? (i.e. wrestling, boxing, etc.) Specify in Medical Chart.   No ___ Yes ___

15. If the answer to question 14 is yes, what is your present weight? ___ kg

    What weight do you intend to compete at? ___ kg

16. Have you ever been refused insurance or been rejected or discharged from a team for medical reasons?   No ___ Yes ___

17. Drug, Food Supplements and Miscellaneous Agents. (List detail for "yes" responses in Medical Chart on page 5.)

    a) Are you taking any medications at present?   No ___ Yes ___

    b) Are you taking any vitamins at present?   No ___ Yes ___

    c) Are you taking any stimulants (benzadrine, amphetamine, etc.)?   No ___ Yes ___

    d) Are you taking any anabolic agents (growth stimulators)?   No ___ Yes ___

    e) Are you taking any sleeping pills?   No ___ Yes ___

    f) Are you taking any other prescription drugs?   No ___ Yes ___

    g) Are you on any non-prescription drugs not listed above?   No ___ Yes ___

    h) Do you smoke?   No ___ Yes ___

A. MEDICAL (Con't)

    i) Do you drink alcoholic beverages?   No ___ Yes ___

    If yes, how much per week? _____

18. Have you ever been advised for medical reasons not to participate in a certain sport(s) for any period whatever?   No ___ Yes ___

19. Do you wear glasses for sports?   No ___ Yes ___

20. Do you wear contact lens for sports?   No ___ Yes ___

21. When was your last chest X-ray?

    Month _____ Year _____

22. When did you last visit a dentist?

    Month _____ Year _____

23. Menstrual and Gynaecology History.

    a) Any menstrual abnormalities, e.g. abnormal bleeding, pain?   No ___ Yes ___

    b) Any vaginal itching or discharge?   No ___ Yes ___

    c) Are you on the Birth Control Pill?   No ___ Yes ___

    d) Any lumps or pain in your breasts?   No ___ Yes ___

    e) Pregnancy? (past or present) (No. of children ___)   No ___ Yes ___

    f) Other gynaecological problems?   No ___ Yes ___

    g) Indicate month and year of your last Pap Test.

    Month _____ Year _____

Confidential When Completed

MEDICAL CHART

DETAILS IN CONNECTION WITH QUESTIONS ANSWERED "YES" UNDER SECTION A. "MEDICAL" ARE TO BE PROVIDED HERE.

Question Number	Date	Name and Address of Physician, Hospital, etc.	Nature of Illness or Injury. Give full details including number of attacks, duration, severity, treatment and results.

TRAUMA CHART

DETAILS IN CONNECTION WITH QUESTIONS ANSWERED "YES" UNDER SECTION B. "TRAUMA" ARE TO BE PROVIDED HERE.

Question Number	Date	Name and Address of Physician, Hospital, etc.	Nature of Injury. Give full details on the cause, date, duration, severity, treatment and results.

Confidential When Completed

513-3B

SPORT MEDICINE COUNCIL OF CANADA
MEDICAL HISTORY INJURY REPORTING SYSTEM

ATHLETE MEDICAL HISTORY PROFILE

To Be Completed by Athlete's Family Physician

PERSONAL DATA:

NAME _____
Surname   Given Name   Initials

MALE ___   FEMALE ___   AGE ___   DATE OF BIRTH _____   SPORT _____
                                                 Month   Day   Year

---

VITAL DATA: Please highlight the athlete's major health problems here following completion of your examination.

_____

_____

_____

_____

_____

_____

_____

_____

MEDICAL HISTORY: This section should be the physician's amplification of the Athlete Health Questionnaire
(513-3A).

1.   ALLERGIES

     Hay Fever   No ___   Yes ___

     Asthma   No ___   Yes ___   Specify _____

     Drugs   No ___   Yes ___   Specify _____

     Others   No ___   Yes ___   Specify _____

2.   MEDICATIONS

     a.   Please list all medications now taken (including injections, Rx and non-Rx).

          _____

          _____

          _____

          _____

     b.   List any drugs taken during the last year.

          _____

          _____

          _____

          _____

3.   ILLNESSES: Please provide a complete history of all illnesses.

     _____

     _____

     _____

     _____

     _____

Confidential When Completed

- 2 -

4. INJURIES: Please list all injuries incurred.

_____
_____
_____
_____
_____
_____
_____

5. OPERATIONS: Please list all operations/surgery undergone.

_____
_____
_____
_____
_____
_____
_____
_____

PHYSICAL EXAMINATION

Temp. ____ F° ____ C°   Height ____ metres ____ cm

Pulse _____   Weight ____ kilograms

Date _____

	Normal	Abnormal	If abnormal, please specify
1. CENTRAL NERVOUS SYSTEM			
a. Reflexes			
b. Proprioception			
c. Balance			
d. Peripheral Sensory			
e. Gait			
f. Strength (gross sensory with manual resistance)			
2. EARS, EYES, NOSE & THROAT			
a. Ears			
(1) Canals			
(2) Drums			
(3) Hearing			
b. Eyes			
(1) Visual Acuity			
(2) Movements			
(3) Fields			
(4) Pupils			
c. Nose			
d. Oropharynx			
(1) Tonsils			
(2) Teeth			
(3) False teeth, please list			
e. Neck			
(1) Thyroid			
(2) Nodes			

Confidential When Completed

- 3 -

	Normal	Abnormal	If abnormal, please specify
3. BREAST EXAM			
4. RESPIRATORY			
a. Lungs			
b. Chest symnetry and wall			
c. Chest auscultation			
d. Chest expansion			
5. CARDIOVASCULAR			
a. Peripheral Pulse			
(1) Character rate: rhythm:			
(2) Carotid			
(3) Radial			
(4) Femoral			
(5) Pedal			
b. Blood Pressure systolic/diastolic			
c. Varicosities			
d. Precardium			
(1) Apex			
(2) Thrills			
(3) Sounds			
(4) Murmurs			
6. ABDOMINAL			
a. Abdomen Wall			
b. Rectal*			

	Present	Not Present	If Present, please specify
c. Tenderness			
d. C.V. Angles			
e. Masses			
f. Inguinal*			

	Normal	Abnormal	If Abnormal, please specify
7. GU			
a. Genitalia			
b. Pelvic Exam*			
8. MUSCULOSKELETAL SYSTEM			
a. Back			
(1) Cervical			
(2) Thoracic			
(3) Lumbar			
(4) Sacral			
(5) Coccyx			
b. Pelvis			

* Optional for youngsters.

Confidential When Completed

- 4 -

	Normal	Abnormal	If Abnormal, please specify
c. Joints - Please examine for pathology, range of motion, swelling, stability, tenderness of each joint and note any abnormalities in the space provided.			
(1) Shoulder - right			
left			
(2) Elbow - right			
- left			
(3) Wrist - right			
- left			
(4) Hand - right			
- left			
(5) Hip - right			
- left			
(6) Knee* - right			
- left			
(7) Ankle - right			
- left			
(8) Foot - right			
- left			
d. Alignment - specify the degree of varus and vagus for the "normal" as well as abnormal alignment condition.			
(1) Knee			
i) varus			
ii) vagus			
iii) recurvatum			
iv) flexion/extension			
(2) Patella			
i) Q angle			
ii) squint			
(3) Tibia			
i) varum			
ii) valgum			
iii) torsion (medial and lateral)			
(4) Foot			
i) pronated			
ii) supinated (cavus)			
(5) Leg Length (true)			
9. SKIN			
a. Bruising or Petechia			
10. MENTAL STATUS			
a. Personality			
b. Mood			

* For jumping and contact sports, please note any meniscal pathology. A standardized knee examination form is attached for detailed analysis of athletes participating in sports in which the knee joint is of major importance.

Confidential When Completed

- 5 -

11. LABORATORY STUDIES

    a. Urinalysis - complete

        (1) S.G. (record time of exam) _____

        (2) Albumin _____

        (3) Glucose _____

        (4) Microscopic _____

    b. Hematology

        (1) Hemoglobin _____

        (2) Hematocrit* _____

        (3) Serum iron* _____

        (4) % Saturation* _____

        (5) Total iron binding capacity* _____

        (6) Serum ferritin _____

        (7) Blood Type _____

        (8) Bleeding/coagulation* _____

        (9) PT and PTT* _____

        (10) Platelets* _____

    c. Blood Chemistry

        (1) SMA 12 _____

        (2) T4* _____

    d. Pelvic Exam (Yearly) Optional for youngsters.

        (1) Cytology _____

* Optional. If indicated.

12. VACCINATIONS

    a. Polio Vaccine _____   Date _____

    b. Tetanus Toxoid _____   Date _____

    c. Other innoculations _____
        (including smallpox if appropriate)

13. OPTIONAL EXAMINATIONS: Dependent on special sport requirements. IF these examinations have been conducted within the last year include copy of report and do not repeat tests.

    a. Chest X-ray _____   Date _____

    b. EEG (if indicated, i.e. boxers) _____

    c. EKG (resting) _____

    d. EKG (stress) _____

    e. Echocardiogram _____

    f. CAT Scan (Boxers only) _____

        NB: Provide Exact Measurements

Confidential When Completed

PROGRESS CHART

New Problems and Ongoing Treatment Records

DATE	INJURY/ILLNESS	TREATMENT

MEDICAL EXAMINATION SUMMARY

FOR THE TEAM PHYSICIAN AND/OR THERAPIST

The confidentiality of medical records will be preserved. The purpose of this summary is to provide details on the athlete's present health status and the treatment program for any injuries to the sport medical and/or paramedical personnel accompanying the team. This summary only and not the complete athlete medical history profile will be released.

Athlete's Name _____ Sport _____

Major Medical Problems: _____

_____

_____

_____

Present Status: _____

_____

_____

_____

Treatment Program for Present Injuries/Illnesses: _____

_____

_____

_____

Limitations: _____

_____

_____

_____

Recommendations: _____

_____

_____

_____

Special Tests: _____

_____

_____

_____

Physician's Name _____

Physician's Address _____

Physician's Telephone No. (   ) _____

Physician's Signature _____

Athlete's Signature _____

Parent/Legal Guardian's Signature _____
(where athlete is not of legal age)

<u>MEDICAL EXAMINATION SUMMARY</u>

<u>FOR THE COACH AND SPORT GOVERNING BODY</u>

The confidentiality of medical records will be preserved. The purpose of this summary is to provide a report for the coaches and NSGB officials regarding the health status of the athlete. By signing this form, the athlete provides authorization to release the summary only.

Athlete's Name _____   Sport _____

<u>Summary of Findings:</u>

Past History: _____

_____

_____

_____

_____

Present Status: _____

_____

_____

_____

_____

Limitations: _____

_____

_____

_____

_____

Recommendations: _____

_____

_____

_____

_____

_____

_____

_____

_____

Physician's Name _____

Physician's Address _____

Physician's Telephone No. (   ) _____

Physician's Signature _____

Athlete's Signature _____

Parent/Legal Guardian's Signature _____
(where athlete is not of legal age)

STANDARD KNEE EXAMINATION FORM

NAME _____ **Date** _____ 19____

KNEE — Chief Complaints:

PHYSICAL EXAMINATION

BODY BUILD: Endomorphic ☐   **Development:**   Hard ☐
               Mesomorphic ☐   Soft ☐
               Ectomorphic ☐   Flabby ☐

HEIGHT _____ WEIGHT _____

ENTERS: Walking _____ Cane _____ Crutches _____ Limp _____

SYMPTOMS: Acute; Chronic; Intermittent _____

RUNNING GAIT: Speed _____ Endurance _____

PAIN: Location _____

        Stop _____ Start _____

        Type _____ Severity _____

        Cutting _____ Pivoting _____ Twisting _____

        Activity related _____ Post-activity _____ Nite _____

JUMPING: Take off _____ Landing _____

SWELLING _____

CATCHING _____

SITTING _____ **ARISING** _____

LOCKING _____ No. Times _____

SQUATTING _____ **KNEELING** _____

POPPING _____

GRINDING _____

LIMITATION OF MOTION: Extension _____ Flexion _____

LOOSE BODY _____

STANDING: _____ Pain _____ Tolerance _____

PATELLAR DISLOCATION   **SUBLUXATION**

WALKING GAIT:

   Level ground _____ Uneven ground _____

   Tolerance _____

   Stairs: Up _____ Down _____ FOF _____ Unable _____

MOTIVATION: Ex _____ Good _____ Fair _____ Poor _____

   Hills: Up _____ Down _____ Give way _____

COMPENSATION: Yes _____ No _____

WEAKNESS _____ **INSTABILITY** _____

LITIGATION: Yes _____ No _____

	RIGHT	LEFT
JOINT LINE TENDERNESS		
Anteromedial		
Mid-medial		
Posteromedial		
Anterolateral		
Mid-lateral		
Posterolateral		
LIGAMENTOUS TENDERNESS		
Medial Capsule		
Tibial Collateral Ligament		
Fibular Collateral Ligament		

	R	L
STANDING ALIGNMENT		
Varus: cms between knees		
Valgus: cms between ankles		
Tibial Torsion: Int. _____ Ext. _____		
Hypertension		
FUNCTIONAL TEST:		
Stationary Jog		
Fast Jog		
Leaning Hop Test		
Squat		
Kneeling		

NAME _____

SCARS: Non-tender,   Non-surgical _____

	RIGHT	LEFT		R	L
PES ANSERINUS TENDERNESS			**MEASUREMENTS:**		
			Leg length _____		
			Mid-calf _____		
PALPABLE OSTEOPHYTES			Mid-patella _____		
A. Femoral ☐ B. Tibial ☐			4.0 cms above patella _____		
			_____ cms above joint		
LIGAMENTOUS LAXITY ON			**KNEE MOTION:** Hypertension _____° to ___		
Forced Valgus at 0° Flexion ___			Extensor Lag		
Forced Valgus at 30° Flexion ___			**PAIN:** On Forced Extension _____		
Forced Varus at 0° Flexion ___			On Forced Flexion _____		
Forced Varus at 30° Flexion ___			On Movement Between _____		
Forced Hyperextension _____			**LIMITED MOTION:** HIP _____ ANKLE ___		
			SWELLING: Intra-articular _____		
ROTARY INSTABILITY TEST			Extra-articular _____		
Internal Rotation _____			**MUSCLE STRENGTH:** Quadriceps _____		
Neutral Rotation _____			(5 to 0) Hamstrings _____		
External Rotation 15 Degrees ___			Hip Flexors _____		
			EXTENSOR MECHANISM:		
POSTERIOR DRAWER SIGN			Quadriceps _____		
			Vastus medialis dysplasia _____		
McMURRAY TEST			Quadriceps tendon _____		
Popping-Pain on Ext. Rotation ___			Patella:		
Popping-Pain on Int. Rotation ___			Height: normal, high; low _____		
			Mobility: normal; increased		
CREPITUS _____			Subluxates; dislocates _____		
			No pain on lateral luxation (45°) _____		
CARTILAGE CLICK _____			Peripatellar ☐ Retropatellar ☐		
			Facet ☐ tenderness _____		
CATCH OR POP _____			Retropatellar grating with ☐		
			without ☐ tenderness _____		
POPLITEAL SPACE			Lateral luxation (sitting) _____		
Posterior Swelling _____			Patellar Tendon _____		
Tumor - Baker's Cyst _____			Anterior Fat Pad _____		
Tenderness _____			Tibial Tubercle: Prominent ☐ Swollen ☐		
			Tender ☐ _____		

X-RAYS: _____

_____

_____

IMPRESSION: _____

_____

_____

_____

INDICATION: _____

_____

_____

513-3C

SPORTS INJURY REPORT

A reportable sport injury is an injury which is sufficient to seek medical/paramedical attention and is in the opinion of the medical/paramedical personnel an injury which will benefit from treatment. MARK THE APPROPRIATE NUMBER CODE IN THE BOX PROVIDED OPPOSITE EACH SUBJECT AREA. ie. Recording Personnel <u>0 1</u>

EVENT _____   DATE _____

SPORT _____   TIME OF INJURY _____
                                                               24 hour clock

INJURY _____

      _____

      _____

HISTORY _____

       _____

       _____

       _____

Recording Personnel

01   Physiotherapist
02   Athletic Therapist, certified
03   Physician
04   other (specify) _____

_____

05   Site
06   Clinic

Occasion

07   Competition, Home
08   Competition, Away
09   Team Travel, vehicle
10   Team Travel, other
11   Locker/Shower
12   Training Room
13   Practice - Warm-up
14   Practice - conditioning
15   Practice - skill training
16   Practice - contest
17   Practice - cool down
18   Residence
19   Horseplay

Sex

20   Male
          Age: _____
21   Female

Home Location

22   rural
23   urban

Status

24   Athlete
25   Coach
26   Official
27   Staff

Level of Athlete

28   Local
29   Provincial
30   National
31   International
32   Years of International
      Experience ____ (specify)

Level of Competition

33   Local
34   Provincial
35   National
36   International

Mechanism of Injury

37   Direct Impact
38   Torsion
39   Stretch
40   Overuse
41   Impingement
42   Shearing
43   Infection
44   Other (specify) _____

_____

Environment

45   Indoor
46   Outdoor

Weather _____

Precipitation _____

Temperature C° _____

Sun _____

Cloud _____

Visibility:

good ___ moderate ___ poor ___

SURFACES

1. Natural Surfaces

   47 Grass
   48 Presc. Athl. Turf
   49 Dirt/Natural Clay
   50 Sand
   51 Treated Clay
   52 Water

2. Artificial Surfaces - Outside

   53 Brand Unknown New*
   54 Brand Unknown Used
   55 Astroturf New*
   56 Astroturf Used
   57 Tartanturf New*
   58 Tartanturf Used
   59 Polyturf
   60 Superturf New*
   61 Superturf Used
   62 Duraturf New*
   63 Duraturf Used
   64 Outdoor Tartan Track New*
   65 Outdoor Tartan Track Used

3. Artificial Surfaces - Inside

   66 Indoor Tartan Surface New*
   67 Indoor Tartan Surface Used
   68 Pro-Gym New*
   69 Pro-Gym Used
   70 Resilient Indoor Surface
           Other New*
   71 Resilient Indoor Surface
           Other Used

4. Mats

   72 Hairfelt
   73 Air Mattress
   74 Foam Scraps
   75 Covered Foam (e.g.
           Ethaloam)
   76 Coated Foam (e.g.
           Ensolite/Resilite)
   77 Urethane Fat Mat (4)
   78 Urethane Fat Mat (8)
   79 Urethane Fat Mat (12)
   80 Urethane Fat Mat (30)

5. Processed Surfaces

   81 Concrete/Tile
   82 Asphalt
   83 Rubberized Asphalt
   84 Cinder
   85 Resilient
   86 Metal
   87 Wood
   88 Portable Floor
   89 Sawdust

6. Snow Conditions

   90 Ice
   91 Wet
   92 New (Powder)

7. Ice

   93 Natural - soft
   94 Artificial - soft
   95 Natural - hard
   96 Artificial - hard
   97 Natural - uneven
   98 Artificial - uneven

Protection of the Body Part When Injured

99 Customary uniform*

_____

_____

_____

100 Taped
101 Brace*   _____
102 Cast
103 Specially Padded
104 Bandaged
105 None
106 Other (specify) _____

_____

_____

*Specify the manufacturer, style, model number and type of all equipment worn.

- 3 -

BODY PARTS

HED	Head	LEG	Leg
FAC	Face	AKL	Ankle
EYE	Eye	FOT	Foot
EAR	Ear	T01	1st Toe
NOS	Nose	T02	2nd Toe
MOU	Mouth	T03	3rd Toe
TEE	Teeth	T04	4th Toe
CSP	Cervical Spine	T05	5th Toe
TSP	Thoracic Spine	SHO	Shoulder
LSP	Lumbar Spine	ARM	Upper Arm
SSP	Sacral Spine	ELB	Elbow
CHE	Chest	FAR	Forearm
ABD	Abdomen	WRI	Wrist
GEN	Genitalia	HAN	Hand
PEL	Pelvis	THU	Thumb
HIP	Hip	IFI	Index Finger
GRO	Groin	MFI	Middle Finger
THI	Thigh	RFI	Ring Finger
NEE	Knee	LFI	Little Finger

TYPE OF INJURY

107	Abscess	131	Fracture, impacted
108	Abrasion	131	Fracture, incomplete
109	Avulsion	132	Fracture, open/compound
110	Blister	133	Hematoma
111	Burn, 1st degree	134	Hemorrhage
112	Burn, 2nd degree	135	Hernia
113	Burn, 3rd degree	136	Infection
114	Bursitis	137	Laceration
115	Calcification	138	Muscle Cramp
116	Callus	139	Occlusion
117	Charleyhorse	140	Other
118	Compression	141	Rash
119	Concussion	142	Rupture
120	Contusion	143	Sprain, 1st degree
121	Corn	144	Sprain, 2nd degree
122	Dislocation	145	Sprain, 3rd degree
123	Edema	146	Strain, 1st degree
124	Embolism	147	Strain, 2nd degree
125	Fracture, closed	148	Strain, 3rd degree
126	Fracture, complete	149	Subluxation
127	Fracture, compression	150	Tear
128	Fracture, displaced	151	Tendonitis
129	Fracture, dislocation	152	Tenosynovitis
130	Fracture, fatigue	153	Unconsciousness

Nature of Injury/Illness

154	New Problem, this season
155	Recurrence, this sport, this season
156	Recurrence, this sport, last season
157	Recurrence, this sport, prior to two years (chronic)
158	Recurrence, other sport, this season
159	Recurrence, other sport, last season
160	Recurrence, other sport, prior to two years (chronic)
161	Complication, this sport, this season
162	Complication, other sport, last season
163	Complication, other sport, since last season

INJURY SPECIFICITY   - Provide detail on the injury. Specify the bone, ligament, tendon, cartilage or muscle injured, i.e. medial collateral ligament of left knee.

_____

_____

_____

- 4 -

FIRST AID TREATMENT

Please specify in space provided.

1.   Ice _____

2.   Compression _____

3.   Elevation _____

4.   Immobilization _____

5.   Wound Closure _____

6.   Stretching _____

7.   CPR _____

8.   Counselling _____

9.   Other _____

10. Action Taken

    a.   no follow-up ____
    b.   referred for medical services ____
    c.   referred for therapy services ____
    d.   hospitalized, less than 24 hours ____
    e.   hospitalized, more than 24 hours ____

MEDICAL TREATMENT

Please specify in space provided.

1.   Activity

    a)   activity not altered _____

    b)   activity modified _____

    c)   rest _____

2.   Medication

    a)   analgesics _____

    b)   anti-inflammatories - oral _____

                       - injectable _____

    c)   antibiotics _____

    d)   muscle relaxants _____

    e)   other _____

3.   Support

    a)   casting _____

    b)   splinting _____

    c)   braces _____

    d)   orthotics _____

    e)   crutches/cane/wheelchair _____

    f)   slings _____

    g)   other _____

- 5 -

4. Surgery - Attach a copy of the operative report for any surgery resulting from a sport injury.

    a)   minor _____

    b)   major _____

5. Reduction

_____

6. Diagnostic Procedures

    a)   X-rays: (i) standard _____

                  (ii) specific - stress _____

                              - arthrogram _____

                              - other _____

    b)   scope _____

    c)   biopsy _____

    d)   lab tests _____

    e)   bone scan _____

    f)   other _____

7. Home Program

_____

8. Referral

    a)   no follow-up _____

    b)   medical _____

    c)   therapy _____

    d)   other _____

PROGRESS NOTES

Date   Remarks

SPORT MEDICINE
COUNCIL OF
CANADA

THERAPY REHABILITATION RECORD

513-3D

MODALITIES

First Aid*	Cryotherapy*	Electrotherapy*	Heat*	Hydro-therapy*	Other*	Exercise*	ASSESSMENT**

First Aid* — First Aid, Support, Strapping, Education/Advice

Cryotherapy* — Massage, Transverse Friction, Mobilization, Traction, Stretching & Flexibility, Other, Chemical Ice Pack, Coolant Spray, Ice Bath, Ice Massage, Ice Pack, Other

Electrotherapy* — Interferential, Muscle Stimulation, Galvanic, Faradic, Neurometer, TNS, Other

Heat* — Hot Pack, Infra-Red, Liniment, Microwave, S.W.D., Other

Hydro-therapy* — Pool, Whirlpool - hot, Whirlpool - cold, Other

Other* — Jobst, Mechanical Traction, Ultrasound, Contrast Bath, Wax Bath, Other

Exercise* — Warm-up, Strength Training, Cardiovascular, Isokinetic, Isotonic, Treadmill, PNF, Bike, Isometric, Other

ASSESSMENT** — By Patient, By Therapist

NAME OF ATHLETE

Rx

Date

* Please specify the type of modality used; the frequency and duration, the type of exercise, etcetera, i.e. ultrasound .5/4

** Assessment: Indicate the state of the athlete's recovery using a scale from one to ten, where zero represents very poor/unable to participate and ten represents the athlete is functioning at 100%. The therapist's assessment of recovery progress and athlete's assessment are to be recorded separately.

CHAPTER

TEN | Monitoring Training

E.W. Banister • H.A. Wenger

RATIONALE FOR MONITORING TRAINING

The importance of planning, implementation, and evaluation for success in sport was emphasized at a Coaching Association of Canada national seminar in 1981. It was suggested that, in order to do well, it is necessary to —

1. evaluate the different physical demands of specific sports at the elite level, and assess national competitiveness and coaching methods vis-à-vis other nations. Assessment of the nature of available support, such as funding, facilities, and services necessary to improve sport, is also an important consideration;

2. plan a program for progress by establishing long-term goals with short-term objectives, and to formulate precise programs to achieve specific objectives. In coaching, it is necessary to establish a three- to five-year major cycle and annual macro-cycles, subdivided into several meso-, mini-, and micro-cycles designed to attain technical, tactical, and physical preparedness;

3. implement flexible, innovative, coaching programs designed to accomplish the objectives, regularly re-evaluating these programs to assess the degree of their success.

It is in the "physical component" of a program where physiological testing may be an important tool to evaluate success and to help in the reappraisal of old programs and in the planning and implementation of new ones designed to achieve as yet unattained objectives.

Although an occasional test or test battery may be useful initially in establishing the status of an athlete at the time of the test, it does little to help in evaluating *progress* resulting from a particular phase of a training program. Established tests under standard conditions must be repeated regularly throughout a particular phase in order to do this. The preceding chapters offer standardized test protocols for valid, reliable, and precise tests, which can be used repeatedly throughout any phase of training to monitor improvement of several physiological attributes. A decision on the exact composition of a test battery is made best by joint consultation between coach, scientist, and athlete.

Data from each test period will add to a developing data base, which permits better interpretation as the frequency with which test and training data accumulate and are jointly analyzed.

MEASURES REQUIRED TO MONITOR TRAINING

Attaining high performance in any athletic event requires optimum interaction of many contributing factors in a complex way. Figure 10.1 shows several, but by no means an exclusive number of, such factors in an overall systems model of performance (Calvert et al., 1976).

Individual physical capabilities, psychomotor performances, biomechanical skills, emotions, and fatigue, as well as actual competitive performances, interact with present training and influence the nature of future training.

Physiological tests measure physical capabilities and are usually used by coach, athlete, and scientist to assist in the evaluation of a particular training regimen; to assess the influence of a particular condition (i.e., nutrition, sleep, travel, etc.) on the physiological state; to prescribe or alter training regimens to maintain strengths and/or to remedy weaknesses; and to evaluate the reasons for success or failure at a particular time. Although the same goals could be used to rationalize the use of testing in other disciplines (e.g., psychology, biomechanics), this section focuses only upon physiology. As the other disciplines formalize and quantify their testing protocols, however, every piece of datum should be integrated into a composite picture to ensure a comprehensive under-

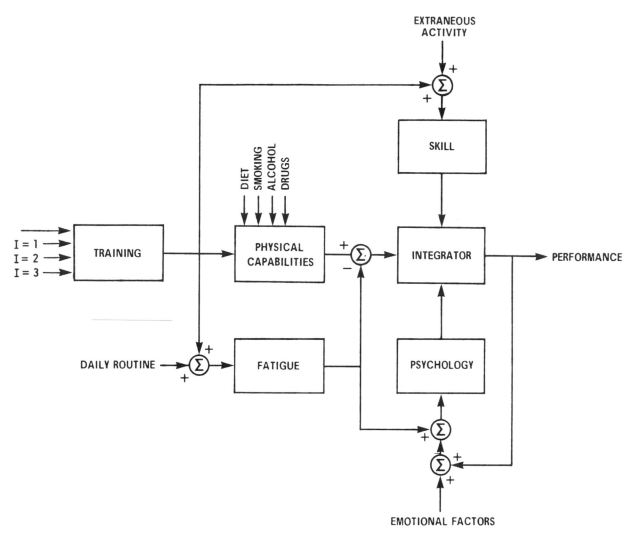

Fig. 10.1 An overall systems model of performance showing the complex interaction of several factors as they contribute to the realization of optimal athletic performance. They range from the influences of common daily life to direct intervention in the organism with training manipulations. The factors also include intangibles such as the psychological effect of a good or bad execution of the performance itself in competition, or even during training. From Calvert et al., 1976

standing of total performance.

This chapter discusses the importance of serial collection, organization, and display of such data in a clearly formatted manner, to monitor and modify the specific training regimens affecting physiological function and competitive performance. Central to this purpose, of course, is the need to quantify not only the physiological results of training but also the training stimulus itself, so that the charting and study of the relationships between the quantity of training (measured in some kind of

arbitrary unit) and the resulting physiological and/ or performance characteristics can be accomplished. In the measurement of certain physiological characteristics outlined in the preceding chapters, a high degree of precision is possible. This same degree of precision is not possible or even necessary for quantitatively analyzing the training stimulus. Whatever measurement is defined for use, however, must still be valid and reliable. In other words, a method for analyzing the training stimulus must be one which measures what it actually purports to measure (i.e., it is valid) and yields similar values when the measurement is undertaken repeatedly and by different observers (i.e., it is reliable).

Systematic analysis of serial measurements of training and physiological function with competitive performances offers some significant benefits:

1. Patterns of training may be distinguished more clearly both between and within different sports. Different methods of training offered by different coaches aimed at the same end result, i.e., winning, may be compared for effectiveness in producing both beneficial physiological changes and superior competitive performance.

2. Injury patterns in relation to training and competition may be studied. Similarly, patterns of therapy, i.e., type, frequency, and duration, may be used to analyze the effectiveness fo rehabilitation programs and thus to enhance the medical and paramedical support of the athlete.

3. Extension of the system to include not only presently carded national athletes but also young, upcoming competitors would result in early identification of ability or deficiency upon which developmental or correctional effort may be concentrated.

4. A wide spectrum of data on the training and current performance of each athlete may be consulted by selection committees and coaches to assist in the decisions at the time of final team selections.

Quantitative Analysis of Training

Although physiological measures of performances may be precise, the amount of training undertaken by an athlete usually is expressed rather vaguely in the comments of the training log book. The inconsistency of writing and the lack of quantification in relating present training to that previously followed are problems.

The first attempts to quantify and record training in a precise way will, of necessity, be arbitrary and subject to change. Gradually, a system will evolve until almost any kind of training may be expressed in a single training unit. An example of such a system has been postulated by Calvert et al. (1976) and by Banister and Calvert (1980). For want of a better term, they have called the unit a Training Impulse, or TRIMP. The training impulse measures the quantity of training absorbed in any given session. It may conveniently be expressed as the product of *stress* (distance run, weight lifted, time spent in an activity) and *strain* (% of maximum heart rate, % of VO_2 max, degree of elevation of the body core temperature, rating of perceived exertion) engendered in an individual by the stress. Thus, stress is the volume of training, and strain is a measure of the relative intensity of that training for an individual. The individuality of this measure is especially noteworthy, particularly where common training is undertaken by a group, since the TRIMP score may be quite different for each individual within the group depending upon the severity of the strain produced in each athlete by the common stress (the communal work-out).

Table 10.1 shows a typical TRIMP calculation for a 6-mile run producing an average heart rate of 130 beats per minute (measured on three separate occasions during the run). Figure 10.2 shows competitive performances of a group of runners, converted to IAAF (International Amateur Athletic

Table 10.1 The calculation of a training impulse score (TRIMP) for a training run of 6 miles at an average heart rate of 70% of maximum.

Athlete's maximal heart rate	= 185 bpm (based on 200 m run)
Average heart rate during training	$= \dfrac{125 + 130 + 135}{3} = 130$ bpm
Training intensity as a fraction of maximal heart rate (strain)	$= \dfrac{\text{Training heart rate}}{\text{Maximal heart rate}} \times 100\%$
	$= \dfrac{130}{185} \times 100\%$
	$= 70\%$
Training volume (stress)	= 6 miles
TRIMP	$= \dfrac{\text{Training Intensity (Strain)} \times \text{Work Volume (Stress)}}{10^*}$
	$= \dfrac{70 \times 6}{10^*}$
	= 42 TRIMP

*The arbitrary division by 10 simply makes the numbers more manageable.

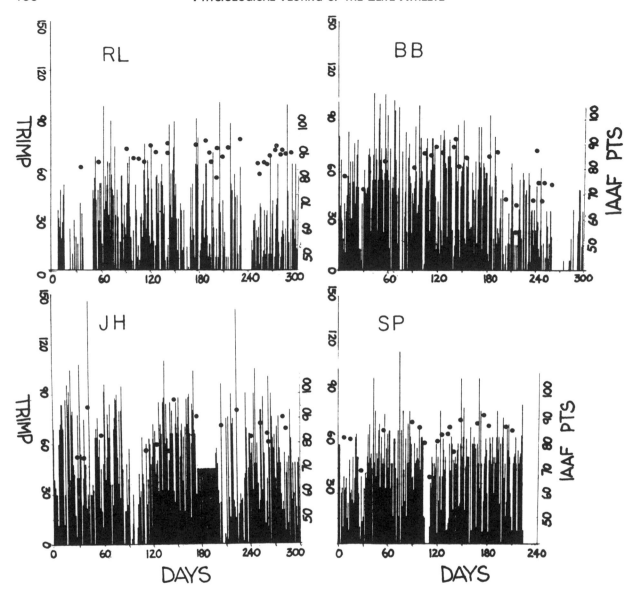

Fig. 10.2   Point scores from competitions (IAAF scores) superimposed upon TRIMP units from training for several competitive runners. It may be observed that there is little coherent pattern to their training, and results over the year changed little.

Federation) points, superimposed on a one-year profile of daily TRIMP scores. It is easy to see that none of these profiles of training produced significant increases in performance between the beginning and the end of the year.

Table 10.2 shows the calculation of an aggregate TRIMP score for mixed training (running and weight training) where weight training is considered not quite as important to running performance as actual running training is. Thus the contribution of the strength TRIMP is set arbitrarily as less contributory to the total TRIMP as running training.

The arbitrary nature of setting up the scoring system (however this may be done) does not alter the quantitative nature of the system or its consistency as long as, once decided upon, the system is not changed. If the methods of scoring

Table 10.2   The calculation of the aggregate TRIMP score for mixed training (running and weight training) performed on the same day

CARDIO-RESPIRATORY TRAINING

Work Volume (Stress)	Average Heart Rate	Heart Rate Intensity (Strain)
6 miles	130 bpm	70%

$$\text{TRIMP} = \frac{\text{Stress} \times \text{Strain}}{10}$$

$$= \frac{6 \times 70}{10}$$

$$= 42 \text{ TRIMP}$$

STRENGTH TRAINING

Work Volume (Stress)	Average Heart Rate	Heart Rate Intensity (Strain)
20,000 pounds	130 bpm	70%

$$\text{TRIMP} = \frac{\text{Stress} \times \text{Strain}}{5,000\dagger \times 10}$$

$$= \frac{20,000 \times 70}{5,000 \times 10}$$

$$= 28 \text{ TRIMP}$$

$$\text{AGGREGATE} = 42 + 28$$

$$= 70 \text{ TRIMP}$$

†Arbitrary divisor for strength training poundage

training are changed, then all previous training must be converted to the new system if it is to be compared to current training.

Figure 10.3 shows a system for running where the stress (volume) of a training session is expressed as one tenth of the duration in minutes of the session, and the strain (intensity) is a number ranging from 6 to 12 arbitrarily aligned to absolute measures of the average heart rate of the session, the per cent of VO_2 max used during the session, or the average speed of running during the session. Two kinds of training are shown, one in which the TRIMP score (quantity of training) is from high intensity, short duration exercise, and the other, from lower intensity, longer duration exercise.

Whatever system is adopted, the daily registration of the TRIMP score presents a visual picture of training upon which all physiological tests and competitive performances may be superimposed.

If the fatiguing effects of training need to be studied, competitive time trials (running) or performance trials (of general application) must be made regularly. If optimal performance trials are desired, then a period of peaking, in order to allow the fatiguing effect of hard training to die away, must be followed before testing begins.

DATA STORAGE, FORMATTING, AND DISPLAY

Precise physiological data collected several times in any period, in conjunction with arbitrarily defined but consistent measures of training, form a data base. This may be continually added to and analyzed, and the results retrieved for display, discussion, and action.

Retrieval of information from the data base and its display in unambiguous form for consideration and interpretation is clearly of prime importance. Several considerations that are relevant to this are —

1 display and communication of those data that have day-to-day or week-to-week importance;

2. display and communication of those data that are of periodic importance, e.g., at the time of team selection, consideration of carded status, etc.

Data that are of daily and weekly importance probably have to do with training and the acute response to the training schedule. Here, quantification of training, quick communication, and turnaround of data collection and display is important. Regular all-out self-testing, regardless of the immediacy of a real competition, is an important feature of the record, allowing a judgment to be made on the extent of developing fatigue. A typical format for display was shown in Figure 10.2.

Consideration of the pattern of training in this way would help both coach and athlete to consider the effectiveness of current training procedures in attaining goals. Comparison of training patterns used by different coaches would enable different rationales of training to be considered objectively, and their effectiveness weighed. Data that are periodic, stemming from the serially applied physiological test, might be displayed as in Figure 10.4. The visual formatting of data in this fashion permits the observer to focus on variables with similar time courses.

Data from several regions can flow into a central

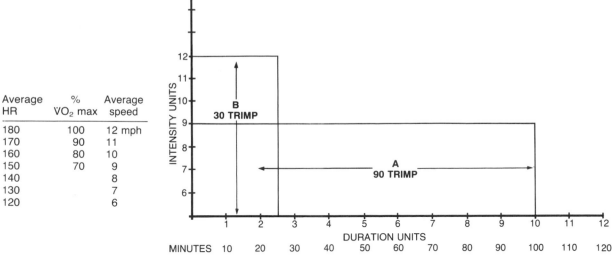

Average HR	% VO$_2$ max	Average speed
180	100	12 mph
170	90	11
160	80	10
150	70	9
140		8
130		7
120		6

Fig. 10.3   A proposed method for charting the dimensions (stress or volume and strain or intensity) of two different training sessions. A: Lower intensity (9 units) over a long duration (10 units). B: Higher intensity (12 units) over a shorter duration (2.5 units). Note the differences in the TRIMP scores (90 vs. 30).

data base and be processed and displayed in two days, if original data are in the appropriate form. Anonymity of individuals may be preserved easily, since athletes could have an identifying number for their data known only to them.

Communicating by postal service or courier, or directly by telephone coupling of standard computer hardware in centers across the country may be arranged. Consideration of cost enters in the final decision.

Data from across all sports could be available to all users of the service for comparison of training plans, enabling alterations toward more successful training patterns. Continuously updated world standards, physiological characteristics of cham-

pions, and competition dates based on a time cycle of a 365-day year would also be a part of the standard format package of the data base system shown in Figure 10.5.

REFERENCES

Banister, E.W. and T.W. Calvert. Planning for future performance: implications for long term training. *Can. J. Appl. Sport Sci.* 5:170-176, 1980.

Calvert, T.W., E.W. Banister, M.V. Savage, and T.M. Bach. A system model of the effects of training on physical performance. *IEE Trans. on Systems, Man and Cybernetics* 6(2):94-102, 1976.

1976 Post Olympic Games Symposium. Coaching Association of Canada, Ottawa.

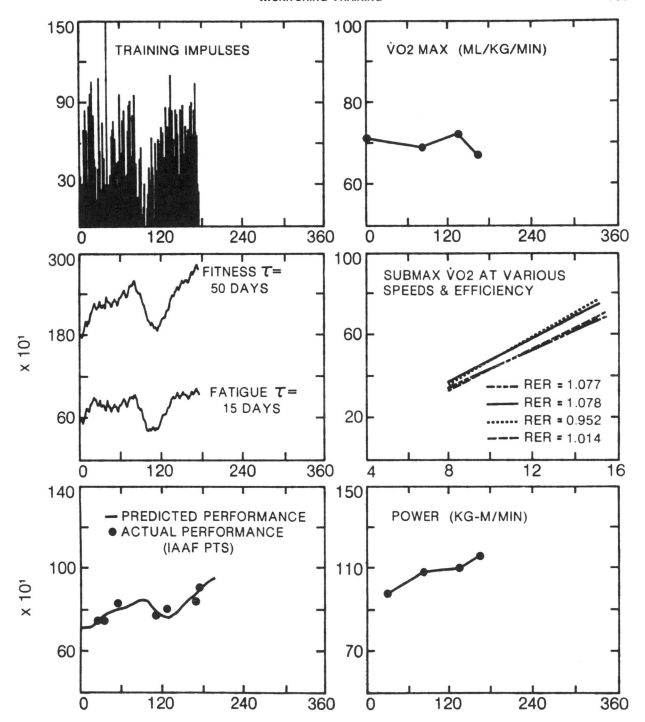

Fig. 10.4 A consolidated display of training, predicted, and actual performance (based on IAAF points), together with some physiological parameters accompanying the real change in overt performance ability.

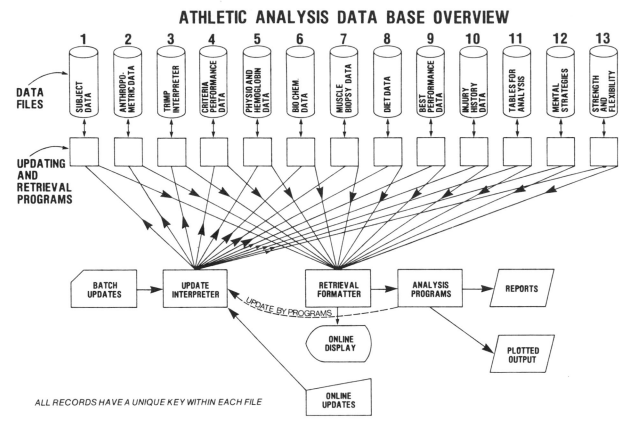

Fig. 10.5   A typical data base system for storage, retrieval, display, and printing of performance and training data in a Performance Monitoring Program.

Index

Letters and digits in brackets following a page number refer to a figure (F), table (T), or appendix (A) on that page.